Selection Criteria for Dental Radiography

Editors: ME Pendlebury, K Horner, KA Eaton

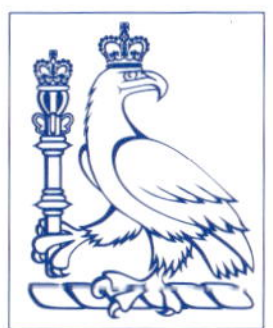

FACULTY OF GENERAL DENTAL PRACTITIONERS (UK)
THE ROYAL COLLEGE OF SURGEONS OF ENGLAND

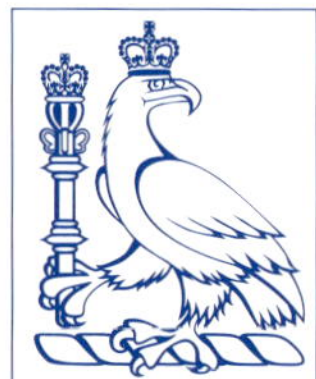

Published by
Faculty of General Dental Practitioners (UK),
The Royal College of Surgeons of England.

Registered Charity No. 212808

35-43 Lincoln's Inn Fields, London WC2A 3PE
Tel: 020 7869 6754
Fax: 020 7869 6765
E-mail: fgdp@rcseng.ac.uk
http://www.rcseng.ac.uk/fgdp/

Selection Criteria for Dental Radiography
Editors: Pendlebury ME, Horner K, Eaton KA

ISBN: 0 9543451 1 8

First edition published 1998
Second edition published 2004

Editorial production: Adèle Moss, Laura Wiles
Design: John Brown
Print management: Publicity Arts, London

Contents

1. Introduction

2. Use of ionising radiation

3.   Radiographs in the management of the developing dentition

4.   Radiographs in dental caries diagnosis

5. Radiographs in periodontal assessment

6. Radiographs in the heavily restored dentition

7. Radiographs in endodontics

8. Radiographs in implantology

9. Good practice

Appendices

Recommendations at a glance

	SELECTION CRITERIA	IN ALL CASES:	SECTION
New Patient		• History and clinical examination before radiographs	9.1
		• Locate and make use of any previous films	9.1
		• Remember: no patient should receive additional radiation dose and risk as part of dental treatment unless there is likely to be a benefit in terms of improved management and outcome of care	2.1
	Dental diseases & growth and development	• 'Screening' radiographs—not indicated	2.2, 3
		• Indicated—dentate: appropriate patient-specific radiographic examinations (see over)	2.2, 3, 4, 5, 6, 7, 8
		• Indicated—edentulous: only when symptomatic, or if area clinically suspicious, or when implantology considered	2.2, 8
Recall Patient	Growth and development	• 'Screening' radiographs—not indicated	3
		• Indicated: use selection criteria	3, 2.2
	High caries risk **Moderate caries risk** **Low caries risk**	• A history and thorough clinical examination is required before considering radiography	4
		• Complimentary diagnostic tools and digital radiography should be considered	4.4
		• Reassess caries risk regularly (in both children and adults)	Appendix 2
		• See *Appendix 1* for radiographic recall intervals recommended according to caries risk status	4.2, 4.3
	Periodontal disease or history of periodontal disease	Patient-specific radiographs should be seen as an adjunct to a clinical examination	5

Review editors

Malcolm E Pendlebury LDS, FDS, FFGDP(UK).
Dental Tutor (Education), FGDP(UK). Adviser in Postgraduate Dental Practice, School of Community Health Sciences, University of Nottingham.

Keith Horner PhD, BChD, MSc, FRCR, FDS, DDR.
Professor of Oral and Maxillofacial Imaging, University of Manchester. Honorary Consultant Dental Radiologist, Central Manchester and Manchester Children's University Hospitals NHS Trust.

Kenneth A Eaton PhD, MSc, BDS, MGDS, MFPH, ILT(M).
Editor of *Primary Dental Care* and *Team in Practice*. Senior Honorary Research Fellow, Eastman Dental Institute, University College London. President of the Education Research Group of the International Association for Dental Research.

Acknowledgements

The editors would like to acknowledge the contributions of the following.

The authors who contributed to the first edition of this publication were contacted and asked to comment on and, wherever they thought necessary, suggest changes to the original text, for which we are most grateful.

We thank Vivian Rushton, Ann Shearer and Paul van der Stelt for their major contributions. Paul van der Stelt was asked contribute in the field of digital radiography, as was Vivian Rushton in the use of panoramic radiography.

Section 5, 'Radiographs in Periodontal Assessment', was contributed by Aradhna Tugnait and Section 8, 'Radiographs in Implantology', by Crawford Grey, reflecting the approach of the European Association for Osseointegration; for these we are very grateful.

We are similarly indebted to NJD (David) Smith, Laetitia Brocklebank, Claudette Christie, Martin Curran, Jon Deeks, Dafydd Evans, Jeremy Grimshaw, Robin Harbour, Peter Hirschmann, Tony Hudson, Chris Longbottom, Helen Marlborough, Brian O'Riordan, Richard

Palmer, Nigel B Pitts, Derek Richards, Pat Rimmer, Judi Rogers, Elizabeth Saunders, Murray Saunders, William Saunders, Ashok Sethi, David Stirrups, and Jeremy Woodcock for their invaluable contributions to this document.

We would also like to acknowledge the expert panel members of the first edition: Nigel B Pitts, Malcolm Pendlebury, Kenneth Eaton, Keith Horner, Alice Keirby, Edwina Kidd, Barry McGonigle, Raj Raja Rayan *OBE*, Chris Stephens, Gail Topping, and Mike Wake. This second edition builds on their work and would not have been possible without their contribution.

Blackwell Publishing are thanked for their permission to reproduce Table 2 (parts a and b) from the European Association for Osseointegration 'Guidelines for the use of diagnostic imaging in implant dentistry'. [Harris D, Buser D, Dula K, Grondahl K, Jacobs R, Leckholm U, *et al*. EAO guidelines for the use of diagnostic imaging in implant dentistry. A consensus workshop organized by the European Association for Osseointegration in Trinity College Dublin. Clin Oral Implants Res. 2002;**13**:566-70.]

The support given for the original project by 3M Dental Care is gratefully acknowledged.

Finally, we thank the following organisations, which were consulted during the development of the first edition of these guidelines.

Anglo-Asian Odontological Group.
British Association for the Study of
  Community Dentistry.
British Association of Dental and
  Maxillofacial Radiology.
British Association of Oral and
  Maxillofacial Surgeons.
British Dental Association.
British Endodontic Society.
British Institute of Radiology.
British Orthodontic Society.
British Society for General Dental Surgery.
British Society for Oral Medicine.
British Society for Restorative Dentistry.
British Society of Dentistry for the Handicapped.
British Society of Paediatric Dentistry.
British Society of Periodontology.

Community Audit Group of Southampton
  Community Dental Services NHS Trust.
Dental Practice Board of England and
  Wales/Dental Practice Division Scotland.
Dental Protection.
European Orthodontic Society.
European Society of Endodontology.
Gerodontic Study Group.
Health Departments of England, Northern Ireland,
  Scotland and Wales.
Medical Defence Union.
National Radiological Protection Board.
Royal College of Physicians and Surgeons
  of Glasgow.
Royal College of Radiologists.
Royal College of Surgeons of Edinburgh.
The Royal College of Surgeons of England.

Preface to the First Edition

The Faculty of General Dental Practitioners (UK) has a declared commitment to 'improving the standards of patient care'. By the provision of standards and guidelines, it aims to help the profession to achieve this goal. Standards and guidelines are simply tools a dentist may use to improve treatment planning and care outcomes.

The *Self Assessment Manual and Standards*, SAMS, published in 1991, is now well known to the profession and has become a frequently quoted source in clinical audit and quality assurance initiatives. Since its publication, the scientific methodology of systematic reviews of the literature has progressed dramatically and this book is based on these developments.

Evidence-based care is well established in medicine and dentistry and these selection criteria and guidelines follow these established protocols by basing advice on the available scientific evidence wherever possible.

This is the first in a series of standards documents from the FGDP(UK) which are based on reviews of the scientific literature and employ the Scottish Intercollegiate Guideline Network (SIGN) methodology for guideline production. They are not constraints but an aid to effective treatment planning and patient care.

I believe you will find this work useful.

Malcolm E Pendlebury,
Dean FGDP(UK).
1998

Preface to the Second Edition

This is the second edition of this work. Several sections have been updated in the light of new evidence and research findings, while others—such as that dealing with the use of digital radiography—have been expanded to reflect an increasing use in general dental practice.

The most important development since the first edition was published is the implementation of the Ionising Radiation (Medical Exposure) Regulations (IRMER) 2000. These regulations increased the emphasis on the justification of any radiographic investigation in order to protect patients from unnecessary exposure to radiation. The regulations specify that the referrer must have specific criteria for the examination even when, as is the case in general dental practice, the referrer and the practitioner are the same person. These selection criteria will form a sound basis for such decisions and so are intended to support practitioners in their clinical work.

Evidence-based care is well established in dentistry and these guidelines were developed using scientific evidence wherever available. The purpose of the publication is a practical one; it is not intended to be limiting or restrictive but to be useful in the decision making process. It may even encourage a change in practice based on scientific evidence.

Editors (second edition):
Malcolm Pendlebury, Keith Horner and Kenneth Eaton.
2004

Introduction

1.1 Remit

These guidelines result from the work of an expert panel, convened by the Faculty of General Dental Practitioners (UK), whose remit was:

> *'To produce selection criteria which are specific to dental radiography. These criteria should encompass all aspects of radiological practice in dentistry, with early attention paid to panoramic radiography'.*

As recommended by the report of the Royal College of Radiologists and the National Radiological Protection Board joint working party,[1] the expert panel focused particularly on primary dental care where the majority of examinations are undertaken.

1.2 Why are guidelines needed?

A useful diagnostic investigation is one where the result—positive or negative—will alter management or add confidence to a clinician's diagnosis and/or treatment planning. When ionising radiation is involved, there is also a need to ensure that any exposure is likely to be of benefit to patients in terms of their clinical management.

At present, there is wide variation in practice relating to when and which radiographs are exposed in primary dental care. There is a need to minimise[1] and/or prevent radiographic examinations:

- Where the results are unlikely to affect patient management and/or prognosis.
- That are repeated unnecessarily.
- That duplicate those taken previously.
- That are inappropriate.
- Where avoidable lapses in quality assurance impact upon patient dose and care.

There is also a need to ensure that, where appropriate, radiographic information contributes to achieving optimal standards of diagnosis and patient care, and that disease is not missed. This may mean that some dentists should undertake more radiographic examinations while others should undertake fewer, depending upon the needs of their individual patients, following history-taking and clinical examination.

A new European Union (EU) guideline on complying with recent EU directives and legislation relating to dental radiography is now available. Its title is *Radiation Protection 136: European Guidelines in Radiation Protection on Dental Radiography*[2] and it provides a set of comprehensive evidence-based guidelines that address the issues relevant to dental radiography raised by European Directives on radiation protection.

1.3 What are guidelines?

Guidelines are systematically developed statements designed to assist the clinician and patient in making decisions about appropriate healthcare for certain specific clinical circumstances.[3]

Just as the term implies, 'guidelines are not a rigid constraint on clinical practice, but a concept of good practice against which the needs of the individual patient can be considered'.[4]

1.4 Why evidence-based guidelines?

There is increasing acceptance in medicine[5] and dentistry[6] that diagnostic and laboratory tests, clinical decisions and clinical practice should all be as 'evidence-based' as possible. This stance is supported by the UK Health Departments[7] and the Royal Colleges[8R] because of lessons learned from clinical treatments that have subsequently been found to be ineffective and costly.

The evidence-based approach is not without problems, including the lack of high quality research evidence in a number of clinical fields. The FGDP(UK) guidelines programme follows the SIGN (Scottish Intercollegiate

Guidelines Network) approach to methodology[9] wherever possible and adapts this, in a pragmatic way, to the particular area under review.

The scientific methodology of systematic reviews has developed dramatically in the last ten years and there are now established and rigorous methods that seek to ensure that the inherent (and often unintended) biases associated with many traditional reviews and professional panels are controlled effectively. SIGN was established in 1993 by the conference of Royal Colleges and their Faculties in Scotland to support the development of national guidelines on a multiprofessional basis. It is now seen as an international leader in this methodology. The key element of such guidelines is explicitly to link recommendations with levels of evidence and best practice for the delivery of patient-centred care.

1.5 Implementation and audit

In order to influence practice positively and be of use to dentists in primary care, guidelines must be turned into useful and usable aids to the provision of clinical care. This can best be done locally at a practice or clinic level.

Using the SIGN methodology and framework, a 'national guideline' is a series of broad statements that relate to the optimal level of care. 'Local guidelines' (protocols) are more detailed developments of these evidence-based broad principles for local application in individual practices.

In order to establish whether the national and local guidelines have had any effect, it is imperative that dentists themselves audit appropriate topics related to their implementation. Suggestions for possible audit topics are set out in Section 9.

1.6 Review of guidelines

The first edition of *Selection Criteria for Dental Radiography*, published in 1998, set out to achieve much at a time when dental services and practices were evolving and when new research evidence was constantly being produced. This second edition is the result of a review of the guidelines:

several sections have been updated in the light of new evidence and research findings and others—such as that dealing with the use of digital radiography—have been expanded to reflect an increasing use in general dental practice.

1.7 Understanding the guidelines

It should be clearly understood that the approach adopted for different sections within this publication has not been uniform. This is because the volume of evidence available for systematic review varies, as does the priority of the topics in terms of balancing risk and benefit. Some sections

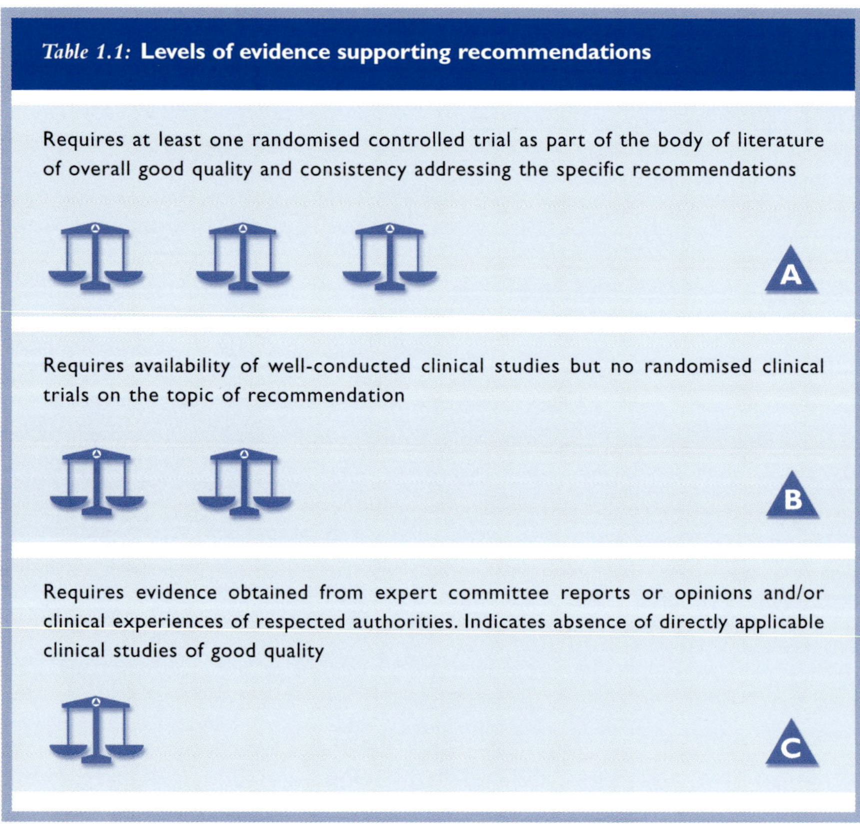

Table 1.1: **Levels of evidence supporting recommendations**

Requires at least one randomised controlled trial as part of the body of literature of overall good quality and consistency addressing the specific recommendations

A

Requires availability of well-conducted clinical studies but no randomised clinical trials on the topic of recommendation

B

Requires evidence obtained from expert committee reports or opinions and/or clinical experiences of respected authorities. Indicates absence of directly applicable clinical studies of good quality

C

include more comprehensive sifting of the evidence, while others rely more heavily on expert opinion and conventional literature review.

The levels of evidence supporting each recommendation within this publication are indicated throughout as shown in *Table 1.1*. This approach is consistent with the SIGN system of classification.[9]

1.8 Guideline methodology

In order to provide guidelines in an evidence-based manner, much time and effort are expended. For the first edition, the subject areas of radiation risk and dose, radiographs taken in children for caries diagnosis and panoramic radiography were identified for special attention, and most time and effort were therefore given to these areas.

- Radiation dose and risk were selected for special attention because they are important issues for both health professionals and patients.
- Radiographs taken in children for caries diagnosis were selected because of the increased radiation risk to this group.
- Panoramic radiography was highlighted as an issue that should receive special attention by the report of a joint working party of the Royal College of Radiologists and the National Radiological Protection Board in 1994.[1]

Since the first edition, further systematic reviews of each topic have been undertaken and incorporated. It is anticipated that when the guidelines are next reviewed, still more systematic reviews of the literature will have been carried out.

The dental literature was searched and appraised in a systematic fashion to produce most of the recommendations made in this publication. References are indicated within the text by superscript numbering, in some cases along with the letter 'R' to indicate that the publication in question is a review article. Where relevant literature could not be identified for review, the authors have attempted to provide recommendations based on 'good practice'/expert opinion, following consultation with specialty groups.

Table 1.2: Review questions

Review question	For all new, recall or emergency patients attending primary dental care:
1	When are radiographs indicated in order that a useful diagnostic yield will be generated in comparison to the conventional clinical examination (with or without assistance from other methods) and thus contribute usefully to individual patient care plans for maintaining and improving dental health?
2	What significant additional age-related risk will follow from exposure to different dental radiographic projections?
3	What evidence exists to influence or support selection criteria by specialty area, in order to contribute usefully to individual patient care plans for maintaining and improving dental health?

At the very least, review questions for each subject area were set (*Table 1.2*). Literature was identified in a systematic manner by accessing electronic databases (Medline, Embase, Index to Scientific & Technical Proceedings, Science Citation Index, and Social Sciences Citation Index). The publications deemed to be relevant to the carefully set review questions were critically appraised and recommendations made from the strongest ones.

The section dealing with radiographs for caries detection in children was produced by the most rigorous methods. A systematic review was carried out in this area, which is detailed in the following section.

1.9 Systematic review of radiographic detection of caries in children

The principal focus on children in this systematic review was adopted for two reasons:

- Risks of ionising radiation are greater in children.
- Most of the available evidence is on children.

In order to produce evidence-based guidelines for the selection criteria for dental radiographs in children for caries diagnosis, a systematic review of the literature was performed. For the purpose of this review, a child is defined as an individual up to the age of 18 years.

A review question was set in order to define the area to be investigated:

For all new, recall or emergency child patients attending in primary dental care, when are radiographs indicated in order that a useful diagnostic yield will be generated in comparison to conventional clinical examination (with or without assistance from other methods), in order to contribute usefully to individual patient care plans for maintaining and improving dental health?

This question was used to produce a search strategy in order to find relevant journal articles from the following sources:

- Electronic databases (Medline, Embase, Index to Scientific & Technical Proceedings, Science Citation Index, and Social Sciences Citation Index). The abstracts of the 115 publications identified in this way were read in order to determine their relevance. Sixty-eight papers were identified which warranted examination of the full text.
- Hand-search of journals up to 1992 (available from a PhD).
- Suggestions from specialty groups.
- 'Grey' literature, such as conference proceedings, dissertations.

The bibliographies of each of the articles identified in this manner were then searched for further relevant articles. In total, 154 papers were identified for first-stage review.

Two individuals independently carried out the appraisal of publications for inclusion in final recommendations; where the reviewers disagreed, discussion took place until a consensus was reached.

The first stage of the review process used a broad 'sieve' questionnaire designed to exclude studies if they were not relevant to the review question, if they were based upon pre-1980 data, or if they had methodological flaws that might contribute an unacceptable level of bias. Following this process, the number of articles was reduced to 126.

<table>
<tr><td colspan="2">Table 1.3: Level of evidence</td></tr>
<tr><td>Level</td><td>Type of evidence</td></tr>
<tr><td>I Low risk of bias</td><td>In vitro validation (study data may be in vivo). Majority of factors in study classified as 'possible bias' than 'probable bias'.</td></tr>
<tr><td>IIa Mild risk of bias</td><td>In vitro validation (study data may be in vivo). Between 33-50% of factors in study classified as 'minimal bias' and more factors must be classified as 'possible bias' than 'probable bias'.</td></tr>
<tr><td>IIb Moderate risk of bias</td><td>In vivo validation. Majority of study factors must be classified as 'minimal bias'.</td></tr>
<tr><td>III High risk of bias</td><td>Research studies not in levels I, or IIa or IIb.</td></tr>
<tr><td>IV</td><td>Evidence obtained from expert committee reports or opinions and/or clinical experience of respected authorities.</td></tr>
<tr><td>Reviews</td><td>High-quality, non-systematic reviews.</td></tr>
</table>

Eighteen of these 126 articles were identified as literature reviews. Ten were accepted as high-quality, non-systematic reviews and another was classified independently by SIGN as a meta-analysis.

A number of factors where bias was likely to be important (in a diagnostic study) were identified and considered for each study. Factors were considered to contribute:

- Minimal bias.
- Possible bias.
- Probable bias.
- Definite bias.

SIGN methodology was refined in order to facilitate its application to dental diagnostic literature (see *Tables 1.3* and *1.4*).

It was on the basis of an unacceptable level of bias that 73 of the primary research papers were excluded from further review. The remaining 35 articles were then graded according to the level of likely bias. The information from each of the 35 articles that had successfully passed each sieve was then graded according to *Table 1.3* and collated in order to make recommendations regarding the exposure of children to dental radiographs for caries diagnosis. The high–quality review articles were also collated in order to assist guideline production.

Once guidelines (or recommendations) were produced from the available evidence, they were each graded according to the evidence that contributed to them in the manner shown in *Table 1.4*.

Table 1.4: **Grading of recommendations**	
Grade	**Recommendation**
A (evidence level I)	Requires at least one study with *in vitro* validation as part of the body of literature of overall good quality and consistency addressing the specific recommendations
B (evidence levels IIa, IIb, III)	Requires availability of well conducted clinical studies but no studies at evidence level I on the topic of recommendation
C (evidence level IV)	Requires evidence from expert committee reports or opinions and/or clinical experience of respected authorities. Indicates absence of directly applicable studies of good quality.
NSR (non-systematic review)	Evidence from high-quality, non-systematic literature reviews in the absence of directly applicable studies of good quality

1.10 Gaps in the evidence

There remain gaps in the evidence; however, the following are suggestions for future research.

- Aspects of periodontology.
- Prevalence of hidden dentine caries (especially in low-prevalence groups).
- Caries-related data of individuals in their early twenties (and older).
- Frequency of review radiographs in endodontics.
- Crown and bridgework radiographs.
- Clinical decision-making.
- Practical caries risk assessment in primary care.
- Symptom-free teeth that are restored—how often do they need radiographs?
- The need for a pre-extraction radiograph.
- Cost-benefit analysis.
- Application of alternatives to radiography for caries detection.

1.11 Overview of recommendations

An overview of the recommendations appears as *Appendix 1*.

1.12 References

1. National Radiological Protection Board (NRPB). *Guidelines on Radiology Standards for Primary Dental Care*. Report by the Royal College of Radiologists and NRPB. Documents of the NRPB: Vol. 5, No. 3. Chilton: NRPB; 1994.

2. European Commission [home page on the Internet]. Brussels: European Commission [updated 2004 March 18; cited 2004 May 11]. *Radiation Protection 136: European Guidelines on Radiation Protection in Dental Radiography*. Available from: http://europa.eu.int/comm/energy/nuclear/radio protection/publication_en.htm

3. Royal College of Radiologists (RCR). *Making the Best Use of a Department of Clinical Radiology: Guidelines for Doctors*. 5th ed. London: RCR; 2003.

4. Royal College of Radiologists (RCR). *Medical Audit in Radiodiagnosis*. London: RCR; 1990.

5. Sackett DL, Rosenberg WMC, Gray JAM, Haynes RB, Richardson WS. Evidence-based medicine: what it is and what it isn't. BMJ. 1996;**312**:71-2.

6. Richards D, Lawrence A. Evidence-based dentistry. Br Dent J. 1995;**179**:270-3.

7. Department of Health. *Research and Development: Towards an Evidence-based Health Service*. London: DH; 1995.

8. [R] Sackett DL, Rosenberg WMC. The need for evidence-based medicine. J R Soc Med. 1995;**88**:620-4.

9. Scottish Intercollegiate Guidelines Network (SIGN). *Clinical Guidelines Criteria for Appraisal for National Use*. Edinburgh: SIGN; 1995.

Use of Ionising Radiation

2.1 Radiation doses and risks in dental practice

2.1.1 Introduction

Radiography is an invaluable tool for the dentist, providing information that is impossible to obtain by clinical examination alone. The importance of radiography is reflected by its frequency. In 1994 an annual estimate of at least 18 million dental radiographic examinations was made for the United Kingdom General Dental Services.[1] Subsequent year-on-year figures show steady increases in radiographic use. Unfortunately, any exposure to x-rays involves some risk of health detriment; consequently, dentists, equipment manufacturers and medical physicists expend considerable effort in trying to keep radiation doses and risks as low as reasonably practicable.

The main value of selection criteria is in reducing the collective dose to the population by eliminating unnecessary or unproductive radiographic examinations.

X-rays are a type of electromagnetic (EM) radiation. EM radiation also includes visible light, radiowaves, microwaves, cosmic radiation and several other varieties of 'rays'. All can be considered as 'packets' of energy, called photons, which have wave properties, including a wavelength and frequency. X-rays are short wavelength, high frequency EM radiation. The importance of this is that high frequency means high energy. When x-rays hit atoms this energy can be transferred, producing ionisation of those atoms.

2.1.2 Radiation damage

An x-ray beam consists of millions of high-energy photons. These can damage atoms in any molecule by ionisation, but damage to the DNA in chromosomes is of particular importance. Most DNA damage is repaired immediately, but rarely a portion of a chromosome may be permanently altered (a mutation). This may lead ultimately to the formation of a tumour. The latent period between exposure to x-rays and the clinical diagnosis of a tumour may be many years. The risk of a tumour being produced by a particular x–ray dose can be estimated; therefore, knowledge of the doses received by radiological techniques is important. While doses and risks for dental radiology are small, a number of epidemiological studies have provided evidence of an increased risk of brain,[2,3] salivary gland[2,4] and thyroid[5,6] tumours for dental radiography.

The effects described above are believed to have no threshold radiation dose below which they will not occur.[7] They can be considered as 'chance' (stochastic) effects, where the magnitude of the risk is proportional to the radiation dose. There are other known damaging effects of radiation (such as cataract formation, skin erythema and effects on fertility) that definitely have threshold doses below which they will not occur. As dental radiography would never exceed these thresholds, except in extraordinary circumstances, these 'deterministic' effects are given no further consideration.

2.1.3 Radiation dose

The terms 'dose' and 'exposure' are widely used but often misunderstood. 'Doses' may be measured for particular tissues or organs (eg skin, eye, bone marrow) or for the whole body, while 'exposure' usually refers to equipment settings (time, mA, kV). In this document, radiation dose is expressed as 'effective dose', measured in units of energy absorption called the Sievert (more usually the microSievert, or µSv, representing one-millionth of a Sievert). Effective dose is calculated for any x-ray technique by measuring the energy absorption in a number of 'key' organs in the body, so that the final figure is a representation of 'whole body' detriment.

Many studies have measured doses of radiation for dental radiography, but only a few have estimated effective dose. There are still a number of radiographic techniques for which no published data are available and some for which very differing results have been reported. In many cases, this reflects controversy about whether salivary glands should be given special weighting in calculation of dose. Furthermore, variation in the technical parameters of the x-ray sets and image receptors used in studies means that care should be taken when comparing dose estimations from different studies.

2.1.4 Factors modifying effective dose

Dose may be profoundly affected by a number of equipment and technique factors, which are detailed below for an intra-oral x-ray set:[8R]

- Kilovoltage.
- Method of x-ray generation (pulsating or constant potential).
- Filtration.
- Collimation.
- 'Cone length' (focus to skin distance—fsd).
- Image receptor (film speed or film/screen speed, or digital system).

In addition to these, there are marked differences in the doses associated with different panoramic machines, principally related to beam slit width and the site of the rotation centres. (Personal Communication. Hewitt JM, Hudson AP. National Radiological Protection Board.)

The many possible permutations of these variables make direct comparison of published studies very difficult. In this document, doses and risks are shown for a typical scenario for intra-oral radiography using a dental x-ray set operated at 65 kV, a 20 cm cylindrical collimator, a 6 cm diameter round beam, and E-speed film.

For practical purposes, doses and risks can be modified using the deliberately rounded multiplication factors given in *Table 2.1* to take into

Table 2.1: **Equipment factors and dose**		
Equipment factors	**Multiplication factor for estimating effective dose**	**Reference number**
Digital system (phosphor plate)	× 0.25-0.75	9
Digital system (CCD)	× 0.5	10
Rectangular collimation	× 0.5	11
F-speed film	× 0.8	12
'DC' constant potential set	× 0.8	13
'Short cone' (10 cm fsd)	× 1.5	11
50 kV set	× 2	11
D-speed film	× 2	14

account your own practical considerations. No account has been made here of the effect of overexposure to compensate for incomplete development; such a practice may lead to considerably higher doses.

For panoramic radiography an assumption is made that rare-earth intensifying screens are in use. Where older calcium tungstate screens are used, doses and risks should be doubled.[8R] Although digital intra-oral systems allow lower radiation doses to be attained, this is not the case for panoramic or cephalometric radiography where there is approximate equivalence between digital and film-based systems.

2.1.5 The risks

Radiation detriment can be considered as the total harm experienced by an irradiated individual. In terms of stochastic effects, this includes the risk of fatal cancer, non-fatal cancer and hereditary effects. The probability of radiation-induced stochastic effects is 7.3×10^{-2} Sv^{-1}. However, hereditary effects are believed to be negligible in dental radiography.[15]

Risk is age-dependent, being highest for the young and least for the elderly. Here, risks are given for the adult patient at 30 years of age. These should be modified using the multiplication factors given in *Table 2.2*. These represent averages for the two sexes; at all ages, risks to females are slightly higher and those to males slightly lower.

Table 2.2: **Risk in relation to age***	
Age group (years)	**Multiplication factor for risk**
<10	× 3
10-20	× 2
20-30	× 1.5
30-50	× 0.5
50-80	× 0.3
80+	negligible risk

Multiplication factor at 30 years = 1

* Derived from International Commission on Radiation Protection Recommendations.[16]

Beyond 80 years of age, the risk becomes negligible because the latent period between x-ray exposure and the clinical presentation of a tumour will probably exceed the lifespan of a patient. In contrast, the tissues of younger people are more radiosensitive and their prospective lifespan is likely to exceed the latent period.

There is often considerable concern about radiography during pregnancy because of possible risk to the fetus. In dental radiography, it is unusual for an x-ray beam to be pointed at the abdomen (only for vertex occlusal radiographs, which are rarely indicated) and, in those cases where this may happen, it is an official guideline to use abdominal lead protection when a fetus lies in the primary beam. While a fetus is at risk of harm if exposed to x-rays, the evidence indicates that fetal doses from scattered radiation during dental radiography of pregnant women approach an immeasurably low level; consequently, normal selection criteria for dental radiography do not need to be influenced by the possibility of a female patient being at any stage of a pregnancy.[1]

Table 2.3 gives doses and risks for the dental radiographic techniques likely to be used in primary dental care. In using it, remember to take into account the effect of equipment differences in your practice, while for risk estimation do not forget to modify the figure according to patient age.

As mentioned, a particular problem arises from the inclusion or exclusion of the salivary glands in the calculation of dose. The salivary glands are not specifically included as an organ in effective dose calculations as described by the International Commission on Radiation Protection.[16] However, in view of the apparent relationship between dental radiography and increased risk of salivary gland tumours,[2,4] many researchers have applied a special weighting factor so that salivary gland doses, that would otherwise be excluded, are incorporated into dose calculation. By following this practice, effective doses and risks are increased.

Despite their principal use in hospital practice, doses for cross-sectional tomography and CT are given because of their increasing use for implant treatment planning by dentists.

From these figures, it can be seen that conventional dental radiography is associated with low doses and risks for the individual patient. However, bearing in mind the large number of radiographs taken by dentists, it is likely that around ten of the estimated 850 fatal cancers attributable to medical radiology in the UK each year (based upon a collective dose of 17,000 manSv and a fatal cancer risk of 5 x 10^{-6}) are related to radiation exposure in dental radiography.

Table 2.3: Effective doses and risks of stochastic effects—tabular summary of literature review

X-ray technique	Effective dose (µSv)	Risk of cancer (per million)	References
Intra-oral radiograph (bitewing/periapical)	1-8.3	0.02-0.6	11, 15,[*] 17,[†] 18,[‡] 19, 20
Anterior maxillary occlusal	8	0.4	19
Panoramic	3.85-30	0.2 -1.9	15,[*] 19, 21, 22, 23, 24
Lateral cephalometric radiograph	1-3[§]	0.34[¶]	25, 26
Cross-sectional tomography (single slice)	1-189	1-14	19, 21, 27, 28
CT scan (mandible)	364-1202	18.2-88	19, 28, 29
CT scan (maxilla)	100-3324	8-242	19, 28, 29

The paper by White[15] represented a recalculation of largely pre-ICRP[16] publications. Only papers subsequent to 1990 are specifically referenced in addition to White. The use of E-speed film and rare-earth intensifying screens has been assumed for intra-oral and panoramic radiography, respectively.

* White excluded salivary glands from consideration in dose and risk estimations, accounting for his lower figures. His figures for intra-oral radiography are derived by halving figures to allow for E-speed film and by dividing original data for full mouth survey by 20.

† Data derived for single intra-oral film by halving figures to allow for E-speed film and by dividing original data for full mouth survey by 19. No adjustment made for high kV (90) used in this study.

‡ Data derived for single intra-oral film by halving figures to allow for E-speed film and by dividing original data for full mouth survey by 19. No adjustment made for high kV (90) used in this study.

§ Figure cited in ref. 26 with no apparent source; however, such a dose figure is compatible with the risk calculated in ref. 25.

¶ Based upon risks to brain, salivary glands and thyroid gland only.

2.1.6 Doses and risks in context

Life is a risky business. Among the many risks to which we are prone, we are all constantly exposed to normal background radiation, which averages about 2200 μSv[1] each year in the UK. Medical exposures (including dental) add around 15% to this figure. With this in mind, a panoramic radiograph may be associated with an effective dose the same as 1–5 days' additional background radiation, while two bitewing radiographs would be equivalent to about one day. For comparative purposes, a chest x-ray (20 μSv)[30] would be equivalent to around three days of additional background radiation. Choosing to radiograph a patient, along with the selection of the technique and its frequency, should be a matter of balancing the risk against the clinical benefits to that patient.

No patient should be expected to receive additional radiation dose and risk as part of a course of dental treatment unless there is likely to be benefit in terms of improved management of the patient. Notwithstanding the already low individual risk, every effort should be made to undertake the radiography at minimum dose to the patient.*

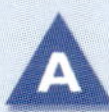

** This important statement is given the highest level of recommendation even though there are no randomised controlled trials to support it. Such a study design would neither be possible nor ethical.*

2.1.7 A worked example estimating dose and risk

All the published work on dose and risk is based upon 'idealised' laboratory studies using phantoms in place of real patients. It is therefore difficult to apply the figures directly to your own practice; however, the following example has some value in demonstrating the impact of relatively simple methods of dose reduction, such as using a faster film.

Suppose you are in a practice using a dental x-ray set operating at 50 kV with a 20 cm cylindrical collimator and D-speed film for intra-oral radiography. You wish to estimate the dose and risk for a bitewing radiograph on a ten-year-old child. Using the dose and risk values in *Table 2.3* and the multiplication factors in *Tables 2.1* and *2.2*:

Effective dose (E) = 1–8.3 μSv,

    x 2 to account for 50 kV set, E = 2–16.6 μSv

    x 2 to account for D-speed film, **E = 4–33.2 μSv**

Risk = 0.02–0.6,

    x 2 to account for 50 kV set, risk = 0.04–1.2 per million

    x 2 to account for D-speed film, **risk = 0.08–2.4 per million**

This example highlights the enormous range of dose and risk that can be found with a single type of dental radiograph.

2.2 The use of panoramic radiography

In the last 20 years, panoramic radiography has become well-established in general dental practice, as evidenced by a seven-fold increase when compared with intra-oral radiography over the same period.[31] As with all radiographic examinations, it is important to strike a balance between the radiation dose received by the patient and the likely diagnostic benefit. Panoramic equipment delivers a wide range of doses to patients and these vary

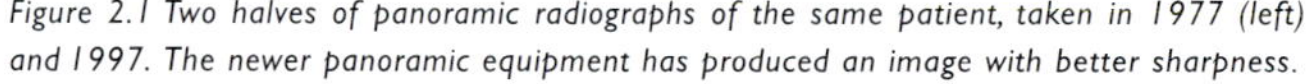

Figure 2.1 Two halves of panoramic radiographs of the same patient, taken in 1977 (left) and 1997. The newer panoramic equipment has produced an image with better sharpness.

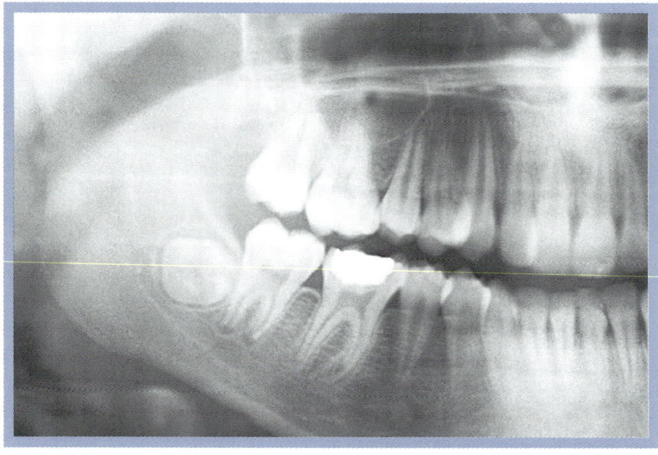

by a factor of 200.[32R] This variability relates to the type of equipment used, as newer panoramic units are more likely to incorporate dose-limiting features. In spite of the undoubted improvements in image quality obtainable with newer equipment (*Figure 2.1*), it is inappropriate to use panoramic tomography as a substitute for intra-oral radiographic examinations.

There is evidence of poor image quality of panoramic films taken in primary dental care.[33] Any faults in the radiograph will inevitably lead to a reduction in the diagnostic value of the examination. It is essential that particular care should be taken in monitoring and maintaining the quality of panoramic radiographs, paying close attention to positioning of the patient and processing. To achieve these standards, it is essential to involve all relevant staff in the monitoring and maintenance of the quality of the panoramic image.

Routine monitoring of panoramic film quality is essential in order to maximise its diagnostic value.*

While there is insufficient research to support a higher grading for this statement, it is a requirement of current legislation.

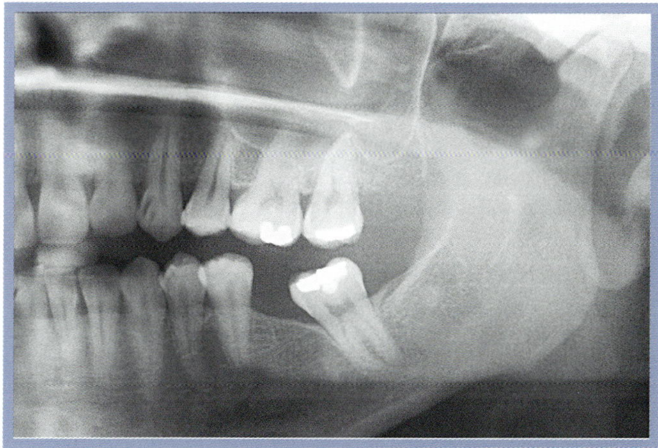

2.2.1 The new patient to the practice

In some centres, it has become routine to take a panoramic film of all new patients. Research has shown that intra-oral (bitewing and periapical) radiography is superior to panoramic radiography for the diagnosis of common dental pathology (caries, periodontal and periapical pathology);[34R,35,36] however, high proportions of practitioners continue to rely on panoramic radiography alone to assess common dental pathosis.[37]

A proportion of practitioners continues to use panoramic radiography routinely to 'screen' the jaws for clinically unsuspected pathology.[37] It is possible that anecdotal evidence of identifying a cyst or other unusual lesion in a patient may reinforce this attitude; however, this standpoint ignores the low prevalence of asymptomatic pathology, and routine radiography without the presence of clinical signs or symptoms cannot be justified.[34R,38] This fact has long been recognised in medical radiological practice, resulting in the cessation of almost all screening practices with the exception of mammography. Recently, the efficacy of mammography has itself been questioned in the light of the findings of a multicentre meta-analysis.[39,40]

It can be argued that a panoramic radiograph may be appropriate for the patient who presents with a grossly neglected mouth, with significant numbers of clinically-determined carious lesions and periapical pathology, along with established periodontal disease (other than simple gingivitis).[41,42] In these cases, it may be expeditious to use panoramic radiography as a means of identifying teeth requiring a more detailed (intra-oral) radiographic examination or, when limited to a hospital setting, prior to dental surgery under general anaesthesia.

2.2.2 The edentulous patient

In the absence of any clinical signs or symptoms, there is no justification for any radiographic examination,[43] unless implant treatment is planned (see Section 8). Where clinical examination identifies the possible presence of an abnormality, such as a possible retained root, then an intra-oral radiograph of the site is the appropriate radiographic examination.

2.2.3 The orthodontic patient (see Section 3)

The panoramic radiograph is used to provide information on the state of the developing dentition and is appropriate when orthodontic treatment is being considered.

Several studies have examined the efficacy of radiography, including panoramic, in orthodontic practice.[44-8] The researchers reported the limited effect of radiography on changing orthodontic diagnosis or treatment plans. Although radiography has an undoubted role in orthodontic practice, such research raises questions about whether the present use of radiography is excessive.

Routine screening of children cannot be justified and the use of selection criteria[48,49] has been found to be effective in determining those children likely to benefit from a radiographic examination.

2.2.4 Prior to oral surgery

The panoramic radiograph (or, alternatively, oblique lateral views) is commonly used to assess third molars prior to their surgical removal but does not need to be carried out at the initial exmination.[50] In the case of mandibular third molars, the radiograph will provide information about the distance to the lower border of the mandible and the course and relationship of the mandibular canal. In those cases in which there is a suggestion of a close relationship of the apices of the lower third molar to the mandibular canal, a second radiograph using different projection geometry should be taken.[50] Routine radiography of unerupted third molars is not recommended.[50]

In other surgical situations, such as apicectomy, root removal or enucleation of small cysts, an intra-oral radiograph may be all that is required for treatment planning.

There is no convincing evidence to support the need for radiography prior to uncomplicated 'routine' extractions in adults; however, where a radiograph already exists, this should be referred to before commencing the procedure.

If extractions are considered in a young child in the deciduous or early mixed stage of dental development, intra-oral radiography is the first choice radiographic examination (or oblique laterals, if patient cooperation is limited). In the older child, if extractions are clinically required and future orthodontic treatment is planned, collimated (field size limited) panoramic or lateral oblique radiographs (as alternatives, if available) are considered appropriate.

Obviously, there will be cases in which a pre-extraction radiograph would be judicious.[51] These are:

- A history of previous difficult extractions.
- A clinical suspicion of unusual anatomy.
- A medical history placing the patient at special risk
- If complications were encountered prior to orthodontic extractions.
- Extraction of teeth or roots that are impacted, buried or likely to have a close relationship to anatomical structures (ie mental/inferior dental nerve, the maxillary antrum and/or tuberosity and the lower border of the mandible).

The type of radiographic examination chosen will obviously reflect the clinical findings.

2.2.5 Trauma

A panoramic radiograph is indispensable when assessing mandibular fractures;[52,53] however, poor panoramic film quality has been shown to severely affect diagnosis.[54] Panoramic radiography has been shown to necessitate supplementary radiography in order accurately to diagnose high condylar fractures.[53,55,56]

If there is clinical evidence of a bony fracture, it is probably more appropriate for a dentist to refer the patient for a complete radiographic examination at the hospital where treatment will be performed. Panoramic radiography has a limited ability to detect mid-facial fractures.

For simple dental trauma, intra-oral radiography will provide greater diagnostic detail.

2.2.6 Temporomandibular joint (TMJ) problems

The panoramic radiograph shows an image of the mandibular condyles and is often used as a first choice imaging technique for those patients with TMJ symptoms. A study[57] of patients with TMJ symptoms found that panoramic radiography provided little or no information that influenced diagnosis or patient management in the majority of cases examined.

The overwhelming majority of patients with symptoms and signs related to the TMJ region are suffering from myofacial pain/dysfunction or internal disc derangements. Condylar abnormality is not seen in the former and only occasionally in the latter.

Radiography is not recommended for patients with joint sounds ('clicking') in the absence of other signs or symptoms.[58,59] Radiographic examination is indicated where there is recent evidence of progressive pathology (recent trauma, change in occlusion, mandibular shift, sensory or motor alterations, change in range of movement).

2.2.7 Suggested selection criteria for panoramic radiography

- Where a bony lesion or unerupted tooth is of a size or position that precludes its complete demonstration on intra-oral radiographs.
- In the case of a grossly neglected mouth, with significant numbers of clinically-determined carious lesions and periapical pathology, along with established periodontal disease (other than simple gingivitis) and where there is pocketing greater than 6 mm in depth.
- For the assessment of wisdom teeth prior to planned surgical intervention. Routine radiography of unerupted third molars is not recommended.

All patients must have a clinical history taken prior to panoramic radiography. When radiographs are clinically indicated, intra-oral radiographs should be considered first because of better detail and lower radiation doses.

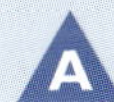

- As part of an orthodontic assessment where there is a clinical need to know the state of the dentition and the presence/absence of teeth. The use of clinical criteria to select patients rather than routine screening of patients is essential (see Section 3).

Panoramic radiographs should only be taken in the presence of specific clinical signs and symptoms. There is no justification for review panoramic radiography at arbitrary time intervals.

2.3 The application of digital radiography

Digital radiography is becoming a more commonly used technique in dentistry. A Norwegian study has indicated that dentists may consider digital imaging when purchasing new radiographic equipment for their dental practice.[60] Digital radiography became available for use in dental clinics in the beginning of the 1980s. Today, several systems for both intra-oral and extra-oral digital radiography are offered by a number of manufacturers.[60-2]

2.3.1 Referral criteria and image quality

Although the technology of digital radiography is fundamentally different from that of conventional film-based imaging, the diagnostic aim is the same. This means that the referral criteria for digital radiography are no different to those defined elsewhere in this document for conventional radiography; however, it is important to know the characteristics of digital sensors in order to understand the factors that may cause inadequate diagnostic quality of radiographs and to be able effectively to correct these shortcomings.

2.3.2 Solid-state sensors

Solid-state sensor systems are built around a special electronic chip consisting of an array of x-ray sensitive elements (called pixels—the abbreviation for 'picture elements'). Solid-state systems are usually known as CCD (charge-coupled device) sensors or CMOS (complementary metal oxide silicon) sensors, depending on the technology used to create the chip.[63R]

The pixels are not only sensitive to x-ray photons but also to light photons.

This makes it possible to add a layer of luminescent crystals on top of the pixels that will produce light when hit by x-ray photons, thus reducing the effective dose of the sensor system. The sensor is connected to the computer by a cable. The electronic information produced by the pixels is transferred through this cable to the computer and stored on hard disk. When the radiographic information needs to be assessed, the pixel data are read from disk and displayed on the computer screen.

The image acquired by means of a solid-state system is available for display a few seconds after the x-ray exposure button has been pressed.

2.3.3 Storage phosphor plate sensors

Storage phosphor plate sensors are based on a different technology. A thin plate of synthetic material is coated with a layer of phosphor crystals. Some of the energy of the x-ray photons is stored into the phosphor layer during a radiographic exposure, producing a latent image into the phosphor layer. The information contained in the plate is released as light photons by exposure to a laser scanner. A photo multiplier captures the light photons; the signal from the photo multiplier is digitised subsequently and stored on the hard disk for immediate or future display on the monitor screen. The scanning procedure takes about 25-30 seconds per image. There are no connecting wires between the storage phosphor plate and the computer, which makes the handling of the plates almost similar to that of conventional films.

2.3.4 Intra-oral systems

Both solid-state sensors and storage phosphor plate sensor systems are available for intra-oral radiographs. The size of the active area of solid-state sensors is usually somewhat smaller than the size of a conventional #2 film (3 x 4 cm); storage phosphor plates have dimensions comparable to those of conventional films. Because of the smaller size of solid-state systems, it is sometimes not possible to show the same area as by means of conventional films, unless an extra image is made. Larger solid-state sensors that approach the size of film are sometimes more difficult to position in a patient's mouth because of the rigidity of the sensor. The cable connecting the sensor to the computer can also impede the positioning of the sensor. Aiming devices for a standardised imaging geometry are available, but usually difficult to handle and semi-disposable. Plastic sleeves around the sensor are used for cross-infection control.[64]

Storage phosphor plate systems, being very similar to conventional film in size and thickness, are easier to manipulate. For several types of phosphor plates, aiming devices designed for film can be used; otherwise, specially designed aiming devices have to be used. The sensor plates are put in a plastic envelope preceding the exposure. Care should be taken to protect the plates from bright light when removing them from the plastic bags, otherwise the latent image will fade and the resulting radiograph show 'noise' and poor contrast.

2.3.5 Extra-oral systems

Extra-oral radiographic machines are also available, based on either the solid-state or the storage phosphor plate technology. Panoramic solid-state sensor systems use a long, narrow array of CCDs to capture an image when the device is rotating. For skull radiography, an array of sensors is used in combination with a narrow slit diaphragm to make the dimensions of the x-ray beam the same as those of the sensor. The diaphragm in front of the patient and the sensor behind the patient's head move at the same speed and parallel to each other, to produce a scanned radiographic image of the object.

Storage phosphor plates can be placed in the same cassettes as used for film-screen imaging (the intensifying screens have to be removed). The phosphor plates are scanned by a laser beam in the same way that intra-oral phosphor plates are read out.

2.3.6 Dose considerations

Dose reduction is often mentioned as a major reason to convert from analogue to digital radiography; however, it is still questionable that digital radiography results in a dose reduction as large as suggested in commercial brochures.[65]

It is true that the dose per radiograph for digital sensor systems is lower than the dose required for conventional film radiography;[66] however, in real practice, the situation is more complicated because several other aspects also contribute to the total dose to the patient. The size of the active surface of solid-state sensors is somewhat smaller than that of conventional film, sometimes requiring more radiographs to be taken in order to obtain the same amount of diagnostic information. Positioning digital intra-oral detectors could be more difficult than positioning film, resulting in more retakes.[67] Because of the ease of taking an extra radiograph and the relatively short period between the exposure and the display of the radiograph, dentists could be inclined to take more radiographs than before. Several studies seem to suggest that this is the case.

The exposure latitude, especially of phosphor plate systems, is extremely wide.[68,69] Although good radiographs can be obtained by exposure times that are about 25% of E-speed film, an exposure time that is four times as large as the standard E-speed time also yields images of good diagnostic quality. Because of this exposure latitude, the user does not get a 'warning' from the appearance of the image when too long an exposure time is applied; thus dentists do not know that they are using a dose that is much higher than strictly required for a diagnostically useful image. Users of digital systems (both storage phosphor plate and solid-state systems) should therefore determine the minimum dose that produces an image of good diagnostic quality. This can be done by taking radiographs of a test object (not a patient) at decreasing exposure settings, until the image quality starts to deteriorate. The next higher exposure is then the minimum (and, in fact, also the maximum) acceptable exposure time.

> The optimum exposure time for digital radiography should be selected carefully. This can be done by making a series of radiographic images at a range of exposure time settings of a test object that is representative for the human jaw, and subsequently selecting the exposure setting that produces the best image of diagnostically relevant details.

  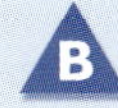

2.3.7 Diagnostic image quality

A large number of studies have demonstrated that the diagnostic quality of digital images can be as good as that of conventional radiographs.[70] Clinicians with considerable experience in interpreting conventional radiographs on a viewing box initially find it difficult to trust themselves when they use digital images on a monitor screen; however, after time, this difficulty should disappear.

The quality of film processing solutions was an important factor for the diagnostic quality of the radiographic image. Similarly, the characteristics of the monitor, and the contrast and brightness settings of the screen are important in digital radiography.[71,72] It is impossible to determine the right exposure time, when the monitor does not show the correct contrast and brightness level. Reflection of bright light sources on the monitor screen should also be avoided.

2.3.8 Comparison of digital and film-based radiography

Several studies have compared the diagnostic performance of conventional film and digital systems for different diagnostic tasks. In general, digital systems are as reliable as traditional radiographs.[73-76,77R,78,79]

The conversion from conventional radiography to a digital system, however, is not a simple and straightforward process. It requires the adoption of new procedures by all members of the dental team and learning new competencies.[80] For instance, in a digital system the radiographs are stored on the hard disk of a computer that is connected to a local area network (LAN). Therefore, the image can only be viewed when there is a computer available that also is connected to the LAN; however, when the computer system is down, the images cannot be accessed.

Nevertheless, there are many advantages in the use of digital films that are not available when conventional films are used. The advantages of digital radiography include:

- Adjustment of contrast and brightness without the need for new exposures.
- Task-specific image enhancement techniques.[81,82]

- Electronic transfer of images to other dentists for second opinion.
- More advanced image-processing techniques, such as digital subtraction radiography.[83R,84]

Because digital radiography does not require the intermediate step of film processing, it is easier to standardise image quality and optimise the quality of the radiographic image according to the diagnostic question that is being considered.[85R]

In this context, it is worthwhile mentioning the possibility of scanning existing radiographs using a flatbed scanner. This technique enables digital storage and display of radiographs without the need for a digital sensor system.[86,87] It also can be used to improve contrast and brightness; however, it does have some limitations.

2.4 References

1. National Radiological Protection Board (NRPB). *Guidelines on Radiology Standards for Primary Dental Care.* Report by the Royal College of Radiologists and NRPB. Documents of the NRPB: Vol. 5, No. 3. Chilton: NRPB; 1994.

2. Preston-Martin, S, White SC. Brain and salivary gland tumors related to prior dental radiography: implications for current practice. J Am Dent Assoc. 1990;**120**:151-8.

3. Longstreth WT, Dennis LK, McGuire VM, Drangsholt MT, Koepsell TD. Epidemiology of intracranial meningioma. Cancer. 1993;**72**:639-48.

4. Horn-Ross PL, Ljung BM, Morrow M. Environmental factors and the risk of salivary gland cancer. Epidemiology. 1997;**8**:411-9.

5. Hallquist A, Hardell L, Degerman A, Wingren G, Boquist L. Medical diagnostic and therapeutic ionizing radiation and the risk for thyroid cancer: a case-control study. Eur J Cancer Prev. 1994;**3**:259-67.

6. Wingren G, Hallquist A, Hardell L. Diagnostic x-ray exposure and female papillary thyroid cancer: a pooled analysis of two Swedish studies. Eur J Cancer Prev. 1997;**6**:550-6.

7. European Commission. *Radiation Protection 125. Low Dose Ionizing Radiation and Cancer Risk.* Proceedings of a scientific seminar; 2000 Nov 9; Luxembourg. Luxembourg: Office for Official Publications of the European Communities; 2001.

8. [R] Horner K, Hirschmann PN. Dose reduction in dental radiography. J Dent 1990;**18**:171-84.

9. FAXIL. *An Evaluation of the Digora Intra-oral Digital Dental System.* Medical Devices Agency Evaluation Report No. MDA/96/01. Norwich: HMSO; 1996.

10. Walker A, Horner K, Czajka J, Shearer AC, Wilson NHF. Quantitative assessment of a new dental imaging system. Br J Radiol. 1991;**64**:529-36.

11. Velders XL, van Aken J, van der Stelt PF. Risk assessment from bitewing radiography. Dentomaxillofac Radiol. 1991;**9**:209-13.

12. Syriopolous K, Velders XL, Sanderink GCH, van der Stelt PF. Sensitometric and clinical evaluation of a new F-speed dental x-ray film. Dentomaxillofac Radiol. 2001;**30**:436-40.

13. McDavid WD, Welander U, Pillai BK, Morris CM. The Intrex—a constant potential x-ray unit for periapical dental radiography. Oral Surg Oral Med Oral Pathol. 1982;**53**:433-6.

14. Silha R. Methods for reducing patient exposure combined with Kodak Ektaspeed dental x-ray film. Dent Radiogr Photogr. 1981;**54**:80-7.

15. White SC. Assessment of radiation risk from dental radiography. Dentomaxillofac Radiol. 1992;**21**:118-26.

16. 1990 Recommendations of the International Commission on Radiological Protection. Ann ICRP. 1991;**21**(1-3):1-201.

17. Avendanio B, Frederiksen NL, Benson BW, Sokolowski TW. Effective dose and risk assessment from detailed narrow beam radiography. Oral Surg Oral Med Oral Pathol Oral Radiol Endod. 1996;**82**:713-9.

18. Cederberg RA, Frederiksen NL, Benson BW, Sokolowski TW. Effect of the geometry of the intra-oral position-indicating device on effective dose. Oral Surg Oral Med Oral Pathol Oral Radiol Endod. 1997;**84**:101-9.

19. Dula K, Mini R, van der Stelt PF, Buser D. The radiographic assessment of implant patients: decision-making criteria. Int J Oral Maxillofac Implants. 2001;**16**:80-9.

20. Gijbels F, Jacobs R, Sanderink G, de Smet E, Nowak B, van Dam J, et al. A comparison of the effective dose from scanography with periapical radiography. Dentomaxillofac Radiol. 2002;**31**:159-63.

21. Frederiksen NL, Benson BW, Sokolowski TW. Effective dose and risk assessment from film tomography used for dental implant diagnostics. Dentomaxillofac Radiol. 1994;**23**:123-7.

22. Lecomber AR, Downes SL, Mokhtari M, Faulkner K. Optimisation of patient doses in programmable dental panoramic radiography. Dentomaxillofac Radiol. 2000;**29**:107-12.

23. Danforth RA, Clark DE. Effective dose from radiation absorbed during a panoramic examination with a new generation machine. Oral Surg Oral Med Oral Pathol Oral Radiol Endod. 2000;**89**:236-43.

24. Lecomber AR, Faulkner K. Dose and risk in dental radiography. Radiat Prot Dosimetry. 1998;**80**:249-52.

25. Isaacson KG, Thom AR, editors. *Orthodontic Radiographs Guidelines (Guidelines for the Use of Radiographs in Clinical Orthodontics)*. 2nd ed. London: British Orthodontic Society; 2001.

26. Maillie HD, Gilda JE. Radiation-induced cancer risk in radiographic cephalometry. Oral Surg Oral Med Oral Pathol. 1993;**75**:631-7.

27. Dula K, Mini R, Lambrecht JT, van der Stelt PF, Schneeberger P, Clemens G, et al. Hypothetical mortality risk associated with spiral tomography of the maxilla and mandible prior to endosseous implant treatment. Eur J Oral Sci. 1997;**105**:123-9.

28. Scaf G, Lurie AG, Mosier KM, Kantor ML, Ramsby GR, Freedman ML. Dosimetry and cost of imaging osseointegrated implants with film-based and computed tomography. Oral Surg Oral Med Oral Pathol Oral Radiol Endod. 1997;**83**:41-8.

29. Frederiksen NL, Benson BW, Sokolowski TW. Effective dose and risk assessment from computed tomography of the maxillofacial complex. Dentomaxillofac Radiol. 1995;**24**:55-8.

30. Myers MJ. Radiation doses. In: Wooton R, editor. *Radiation Protection of Patients*. Cambridge: Cambridge University Press; 1993.

31. Dental Practice Board (DPB) for England and Wales. *Dental Data Services. Radiographic Examinations 1981-2001*. Eastbourne: DPB; 2002.

32. [R] Napier ID. Reference doses for dental radiography. Br Dent J. 1999;**186**:392-6.

33. Rushton VE, Horner K, Worthington HM. The quality of panoramic radiographs in general dental practice. Br Dent J. 1999;**186**:630-3.

34. [R] Rushton VE, Horner K. The use of panoramic radiology in dental practice. J Dent. 1996;**24**:185-201.

35. Thomas MF, Ricketts DNJ, Wilson RF. Occlusal caries diagnosis in molar teeth from bitewing and panoramic radiographs. Prim Dent Care. 2001;**8**:63-9.

36. Pepelassi EA, Diamanti-Kipioti A. Selection of the most accurate method of conventional radiography for the assessment of periodontal osseous destruction. J Clin Periodontol. 1997;**24**:557-67.

37. Rushton VE, Horner K, Worthington HV. Screening panoramic radiology of adults in general dental practice: radiological findings. Br Dent J. 2001;**190**:495-501.

38. Richardson PS. Selective periapical radiology compared to panoramic screening. Prim Dent Care. 1997;**4**:95-9.

39. Gotzsche PC, Olsen O. Is screening for breast cancer with mammography justifiable? Lancet. 2000;**355**:129-34.

40. Gotzsche PC. Debate on screening for breast cancer is not over. BMJ. 2001;**323**:693.

41. Rushton VE, Horner K, Worthington HM. Screening panoramic radiography of new adult patients in general dental practice: diagnostic yield when combined with bitewing radiography and identification of selection criteria. Br Dent J. 2002;**192**:275-9.

42. Rushton VE, Horner K, Worthington HM. Screening panoramic radiography of new adult patients in general dental practice: a measurement of diagnostic yield of relevance to treatment and identification of selection criteria. Oral Surg Oral Med Oral Pathol Oral Radiol Endod. 2002;**93**:488-95.

43. Bohay RN, Stephens RG, Kogon SL. A study of the impact of screening or selective radiography on the treatment and post delivery outcome for edentulous patients. Oral Surg Oral Med Oral Pathol Oral Radiol Endod. 1998;**86**:353-9.

44. Atchinson KA. Radiographic examinations of orthodontic educators and practitioners. J Dent Educ 1986;**50**:651-5.

45. Bruks A, Enberg K, Nordqvist I, Hansson AS, Jansson L, Svenson B. Radiographic examinations as an aid to orthodontic diagnosis and treatment planning. Swed Dent J. 1999;**23**:77-85.

46. Han UK, Vig KWL, Weintraud JA, Vig PS, Kowalski CJ. Consistency of orthodontic treatment decisions relative to diagnostic records. Am J Orthop Dentofac Orthop. 1991;**100**:212-9.

47. Atchinson KA, Luke LS, White SC. Contribution of pretreatment radiographs to orthodontists' decision making. Oral Surg Oral Med Oral Pathol. 1991;**71**:238-45.

48. Atchinson KA, Luke LS, White SC. An algorithm for ordering pretreatment orthodontic radiographs. Am J Orthod Dentofac Orthop. 1992;**102**:29-44.

49. Hintze H, Wenzel A, Williams S. Diagnostic value of clinical examination for the identification of children in need of orthodontic treatment compared with clinical examination and screening pantomography. Eur J Orthod. 1990;**12**:385-8.

50. Scottish Intercollegiate Guidelines Network (SIGN). Management of Unerupted and Impacted Third Molar Teeth. SIGN publication no 43. Edinburgh: SIGN; 2000.

51. Dental Protection. The whole tooth—and nothing but the tooth! Dent News. 1999;**20**:7-8.

52. Guss DA, Clark RF, Peitz T, Taub M. Pantomography vs mandibular series for the detection of mandibular fractures. Acad Emerg Med. 2000;**7**:141-5.

53. Nair MK, Nair UP. Imaging of mandibular trauma: ROC analysis. Acad Emerg Med. 2001;**8**:689-95.

54. Markowitz BL, Sinow JD, Kawamoto HK Jr, Shewmake K, Khoumehr F. Prospective comparison of axial computed tomography and standard and panoramic radiographs in the diagnosis of mandibular fractures. Ann Plast Surg. 1999;**42**:163-9.

55. Wilson IF, Lokeh A, Benjamin CI, Hilger PA, Hamler DD, Ondrey FG, et al. Contribution of conventional axial computed tomography (nonhelical), in conjunction with panoramic tomography (zonography), in evaluating mandibular fractures. Ann Plast Surg. 2000;**45**:415-21.

56. Schimming R, Eckelt U, Kittner T. The value of computer tomograms in fractures of the mandibular condylar process. Oral Surg Oral Med Oral Pathol Oral Radiol Endod. 1999;**87**:632-9.

57. Epstein JB, Caldwell J, Black G. The utility of panoramic imaging of the temporomandibular joint in patients with temporomandibular disorders. Oral Surg Oral Med Oral Pathol Oral Radiol Endod. 2001;**92**:236-9.

58. McNeill C, Mohl ND, Rugh JD, Tanaka TT. Temporomandibular disorders: diagnosis, management, education, and research. J Am Dent Assoc. 1990;**120**:253-63.

59. Brooks SL, Brand JW, Gibbs SJ, Hollender L, Lurie AG, Omnell K-A, et al. Imaging of the temporomandibular joint: a position paper of the American Academy of Oral and Maxillofacial Radiology. Oral Surg Oral Med Oral Pathol Oral Radiol Endod. 1997;**83**:609-18.

60. Miles DA, Razzano MR. The future of digital imaging in dentistry. Dent Clin North Am. 2000;**44**:427-38.

61. van der Stelt PF. Principles of digital imaging. Dent Clin North Am. 2000;**44**:237-48.

62. Sanderink GC, Miles DA. Intra-oral detectors. CCD, CMOS, TFT, and other devices. Dent Clin North Am. 2000;**44**:249-55.

63. [R] Wenzel A, Grondahl HG. Direct digital radiography in the dental office. Int Dent J. 1995;**45**:27-34.

64. Wenzel A, Frandsen E, Hintze H. Patient discomfort and cross-infection control in bitewing examination with a storage phosphor plate and a CCD-based sensor. J Dent. 1999;**27**:243-6.

65. Velders XL, Sanderink GC, van der Stelt PF. Dose reduction of two digital sensor systems measuring file lengths. Oral Surg Oral Med Oral Pathol Oral Radiol Endod. 1996;**81**:607-12.

66. Dula K, Sanderink G, van der Stelt PF, Mini R, Buser D. Effects of dose reduction on the detectability of standardized radiolucent lesions in digital panoramic radiography. Oral Surg Oral Med Oral Pathol Oral Radiol Endod. 1998;**86**:227-33.

67. Versteeg CH, Sanderink GC, van Ginkel FC, van der Stelt PF. An evaluation of periapical radiography with a charge-coupled device. Dentomaxillofac Radiol. 1998;**27**:97-101.

68. Borg E, Grondahl HG. On the dynamic range of different X-ray photon detectors in intra-oral radiography. A comparison of image quality in film, charge-coupled device and storage phosphor systems. Dentomaxillofac Radiol. 1996;**25**:82-8.

69. Borg E, Attaelmanan A, Grondahl HG. Subjective image quality of solid-state and photostimulable phosphor systems for digital intra-oral radiography. Dentomaxillofac Radiol. 2000;**29**:70-5.

70. Huda W, Rill LN, Benn DK, Pettigrew JC. Comparison of a photostimulable phosphor system with film for dental radiology. Oral Surg Oral Med Oral Pathol Oral Radiol Endod. 1997;**83**:725-31.

71. Versteeg CH, Sanderink GC, Lobach SR, van der Stelt PF. Reduction in size of digital images: does it lead to less detectability or loss of diagnostic information? Dentomaxillofac Radiol. 1998;**27**:93-6.

72. Møystad A, Svanaes DB, Larheim TA, Grondahl HG. The effect of cathode ray tube display format on observer performance in dental digitized radiography: comparison with plain films. Dentomaxillofac Radiol. 1994;**23**:206-10.

73. Syriopoulos K, Sanderink GC, Velders XL, van der Stelt PF. Radiographic detection of approximal caries: a comparison of dental films and digital imaging systems. Dentomaxillofac Radiol. 2000;**29**:312-8.

74. Borg E, Kallqvist A, Grondahl K, Grondahl HG. Film and digital radiography for detection of simulated root resorption cavities. Oral Surg Oral Med Oral Pathol Oral Radiol Endod. 1998;**86**:110-4.

75. Borg E, Grondahl HG. Endodontic measurements in digital radiographs acquired by a photostimulable, storage phosphor system. Endod Dent Traumatol. 1996;**12**:20-4.

76. Hintze H, Wenzel A, Frydenberg M. Accuracy of caries detection with four storage phosphor systems and E-speed radiographs. Dentomaxillofac Radiol. 2002;**31**:170-5.

77. [R] Wenzel A. Digital imaging for dental caries. Dent Clin North Am. 2000;**44**:319-38.

78. Borg E. Some characteristics of solid-state and photo-stimulable phosphor detectors for intra-oral radiography. Swed Dent J Suppl. 1999;**139**:i-viii, 1-67.

79. Abreu M Jr, Mol A, Ludlow JB. Performance of RVGui sensor and Kodak Ektaspeed Plus film for proximal caries detection. Oral Surg Oral Med Oral Pathol Oral Radiol Endod. 2001;**91**:381-5.

80. Berkhout WE, Sanderink GC, Van der Stelt PF. A comparison of digital and film radiography in Dutch dental practices assessed by questionnaire. Dentomaxillofac Radiol. 2002;**31**:93-9.

81. Møystad A, Svanaes DB, Risnes S, Larheim TA, Grondahl HG. Detection of approximal caries with a storage phosphor system. A comparison of enhanced digital images with dental X-ray film. Dentomaxillofac Radiol. 1996;**25**:202-6.

82. Gotfredsen E, Wenzel A, Grondahl HG. Observers' use of image enhancement in assessing caries in radiographs taken by four intra-oral digital systems. Dentomaxillofac Radiol. 1996;**25**:34-8.

83. [R] Mol A. Image processing tools for dental applications. Dent Clin North Am. 2000;**44**:299-318.

84. Mol A, Dunn SM, van der Stelt PF. Diagnosing periapical bone lesions on radiographs by means of texture analysis. Oral Surg Oral Med Oral Pathol. 1992;**73**:746-50.

85. [R] Versteeg CH, Sanderink GC, van der Stelt PF. Efficacy of digital intra-oral radiography in clinical dentistry. J Dent. 1997;**25**:215-24.

86. Attaelmanan A, Borg E, Grondahl HG. Digitisation and display of intra-oral films. Dentomaxillofac Radiol. 2000;**29**:97-102.

87. Janhom A, van Ginkel FC, van Amerongen JP, van der Stelt PF. Scanning resolution and the detection of approximal caries. Dentomaxillofac Radiol. 2001;**30**:166-71.

Radiographs in the Management of the Developing Dentition

3.1 Introduction

A high proportion of the child population eventually seeks orthodontic treatment. Most of those who need this are appropriately treated at around 12-13 years of age and require radiographs to confirm the presence and condition of all teeth as an aid to treatment planning. A few children may need radiographs before this time; for instance, in cases where there is:

- Variation from normal development.
- Dental pain.
- Trauma.

In children it is particularly important that radiation dosage is kept as low as possible.

There is no scientific evidence to support any claimed benefit from radiographic screening for the purpose of assessing malocclusion and timing of treatment.[1-3]

> The patient must have a history taken and be examined clinically prior to the taking of any orthodontic radiograph to ensure that appropriate views are taken.

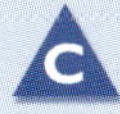

3.2 Type of radiograph

Usually the radiographic investigation will consist of a dental panoramic tomograph[4] or left and right rotated oblique lateral (bimolar) views.[5] An upper anterior occlusal view may be required to supplement rotated oblique lateral films. Multiple intra-oral films to check for the presence of successional teeth cannot be justified.

Rare-earth intensifying screens significantly reduce radiation without affecting the diagnostic yield.[6R] Similarly, where available, selective collimation ('child setting') permits significant dose reductions.

Where a dental panoramic tomograph is available, an anterior occlusal film may be indicated where:

- An examination of the anterior teeth suggests the presence of an abnormality.
- An abnormality is found on examination of the panoramic film.
- Localisation of unerupted teeth is to be carried out using parallax techniques.[7,8]

Examples include:

- Suggestion of a supernumerary tooth.
- Misplaced unerupted canines.

A periapical film may be indicated when the clinical examination of the incisors suggests an abnormality.[9,10] Where dental panoramic tomography is used, an anterior occlusal film may be justified in the case of abnormal incisor relationships. This is particularly important if there is a clinical indication for doubting the condition of the anterior teeth; however, even here a periapical film may be more reliable.

3.3 Clinical indications

Full radiographic examination is rarely justified in children below eight years of age. Radiographs may be indicated in the circumstances outlined below.

3.3.1 Abnormalities

Radiographs may be indicated when the clinical examination leaves reasonable suspicion as to the presence of an abnormality that may affect dentofacial development. There are cases that may benefit from the taking of radiographs for occlusal management purposes before the age at which a full orthodontic assessment can be made, including those where there is:

- A history of hypodontia.
- A history of trauma.
- An unusual eruption pattern.
- Delayed appearance of teeth or unexplained missing teeth.
- A clinically impacted tooth/teeth.
- Unusual tooth morphology.
- Unexplained hard dentoalveolar swelling.
- Mobility of teeth.
- First molars of poor long-term prognosis.

3.3.2 Enforced extractions

Radiographs are indicated when extractions are required to maintain oral health. It is important to consider the presence, position and development of the successional teeth. Specialist advice may be necessary to plan possible compensating and/or balancing extractions.

Careful planning at this stage could simplify future orthodontic management. The information gained from these radiographs may be sufficient for planning orthodontic treatment. When referring a patient to a specialist orthodontist, these films must be made available to avoid any unnecessary duplication.

3.3.3 A child new to the practice

The routine taking of radiographs for a new patient is not acceptable clinical practice. Any radiographs taken of a new patient must follow a clinical examination and appropriate justification. Every effort should be made to obtain any radiographs from the previous practitioner.

Where earlier radiographs have been taken at another practice, efforts should be made to obtain these.

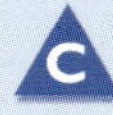

3.3.4 Referral for orthodontic treatment

When a patient is to be referred for specialist treatment, it is only necessary to take those radiographs required to make this decision. Care should be taken to ensure that these and any other relevant films are forwarded.

Where previous radiographs are available, further films should only be taken if earlier views cannot be obtained or no longer provide sufficient information for the appropriate clinical management of the patient.

To reduce the instances of repeat radiography, practitioners referring and accepting patients for orthodontic treatment should develop local agreements over the forwarding and/or copying of films. The increased availability of digital images may facilitate this process.

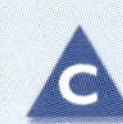

3.4 Orthodontic assessment

As a general guide, orthodontic radiographs are most likely to be needed for children aged 10-14 years. At this age, the deciduous dentition is changing to the permanent dentition and orthodontic treatment may be necessary.

Radiographs are essential when orthodontic extractions are being considered and deciduous teeth are still present in the mouth. They are also indicated when deciduous teeth are retained past their normal shedding date and there is a possibility of absent permanent teeth or displaced teeth such as upper permanent canines.

In the adolescent patient, when all successional teeth have erupted, radiographs may not be necessary to formulate a treatment plan. Recent research has shown that a clinical examination, supplemented by study models, may provide adequate information.[11,12]

Before any orthodontic radiographs are taken, adult patients should receive a clear explanation of what orthodontic treatment would involve.

It is unnecessary to take pretreatment orthodontic radiographs solely for medicolegal reasons.

Cephalometric radiographs are likely to be needed only in a specialist practice or in a practice with a high proportion of orthodontic patients under treatment. The indications are mainly for patients with a skeletal discrepancy who will require two arch-fixed appliances or functional appliance treatment.

Where cephalometric radiographs are required for the assessment of skeletal discrepancy, the greatest value will be obtained if these are traced or digitised.

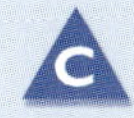

There is no evidence that a single true lateral cephalometric skull radiograph is of use in the prediction of facial growth and films should not be taken for this purpose.

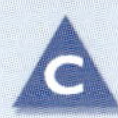

Posterior-anterior (PA) skull views may be of use in those patients presenting with facial asymmetry and may occasionally be helpful in the assessment of certain jaw or dental anomalies.

There are very few indications for a vertex occlusal view in any patient and, if this view is employed, intensifying screens/cassette must be used.

More detailed information is contained in the British Orthodontic Society's *Orthodontic Radiographs Guidelines.*[9]

3.5 Monitoring treatment

Given that the radiation dosage should always be kept as low as possible, radiographic monitoring of treatment progress can only be justified in certain circumstances.

In certain types of treatment, for example in the management of unerupted teeth, radiographs may be the only means of assessing progress. Usually these will take the form of a repeat intra-oral film to assess that a tooth is erupting or that it is causing no damage to adjacent teeth.

3.5.1 Treatment progress

Occasionally it may be necessary to expose additional radiographs during treatment when an abnormal or unexpected response to orthodontic tooth movement is suspected, for example an increased risk of root resorption or abnormal mobility. These are most likely to be intra-oral films, which will ensure maximum information.

Standard occlusal views may be indicated 6-9 months after the start of fixed appliance treatment to check on root resorption if a tooth becomes excessively mobile.

Where fixed appliances in both arches and/or functional appliances are being used, a cephalometric record may be necessary in order to monitor progress.

Skeletal discrepancy problems that require correction by a combination of orthodontic and surgical approach often require progress radiographs. These are necessary to determine whether presurgical targets have been met and to allow final surgical planning.

3.5.2 Completion of treatment

Radiographs are rarely indicated at this stage; however, if the clinical condition gives cause for concern at the completion of treatment, appropriate radiographs may be necessary to help plan the retention regimen. The need for such radiographs must be clearly explained to the patient or parent.

Current guidelines on the management of third molars suggest that there is no indication for the radiographic assessment of these teeth at the completion of orthodontic treatment.[8]

3.6 References

1. Hintze H, Wenzel A, Williams S. Diagnostic value of clinical examination for the identification of children in need of orthodontic treatment compared with clinical examination and screening pantomography. Eur J Orthod. 1990;**12**:385-8.

2. Hintze H, Wenzel A. Oral radiographic screening in Danish schoolchildren. Scand J Dent Res. 1990;**98**:47-52.

3. Wenzel A. Radiographic screening for identification of children in need of orthodontic treatment [editorial]. Dentomaxillofac Radiol. 1991;**20**:115-6.

4. Neal JJ, Bowden D. The diagnostic value of panoramic tomography in children aged 9 to 10 years. Br J Orthod. 1988;**15**:193-7.

5. Osman F, Davies RM, Stephens CD, Dowell TB. Radiographs taken for orthodontic purposes in general practice. Br J Orthod. 1985;**12**:82-6.

6. [R] Taylor TS, Ackerman RJ, Hardman PK. Exposure reduction and image quality in orthodontic radiology: a review of the literature. Am J Orthod Dentofac Orthop. 1988;**93**:68-77.

7. Southall PJ, Gravely J. Radiographic localisation of unerupted teeth in the anterior part of the maxilla. Br J Orthod. 1987;**14**:235-43.

8. Faculty of Dental Surgery. *The Management of Patients with Third Molar Teeth*. Report of a Working Party convened by the Faculty of Dental Surgery, The Royal College of Surgeons of England. London: Faculty of Dental Surgery RCS (Eng); 1997.

9. Isaacson KG, Thom AR, editors. *Orthodontic Radiographs Guidelines (Guidelines for the Use of Radiographs in Clinical Orthodontics)*. 2nd ed. London: British Orthodontic Society; 2001.

10. Ferguson JW, Evans RJW, Cheng LHH. Diagnostic accuracy and observer performance in the diagnosis of abnormalities of the anterior maxilla: a comparison of panoramic with intra-oral radiography. Br Dent J. 1992;**173**:265-71.

11. Taylor NG, Jones AG. Are anterior occlusal radiographs indicated to supplement panoramic radiography during orthodontic assessment? Br Dent J. 1995;**179**:377-81.

12. Brucks A, Enberg K, Nordqvist I, Hansson AS, Jansson I, Svenson, B. Radiographic examinations as an aid to orthodontic diagnosis and treatment planning. Swed Dent J. 1999;**23**:77-85.

Radiographs in Dental Caries Diagnosis

4.1 Introduction

Most of the available research on radiographic diagnosis of dental caries concerns children. This may be because of the greater risks of ionising radiation in children and the prevalence of caries in younger individuals. For these reasons, children were selected as a principal focus within this section of the guidelines. The rigorous methodology used to derive the recommendations that follow can be examined in Section 2.

When assessing caries risk, clinicians should note that in 2003/2004 the Guideline Development Group and the National Institute for Clinical Excellence (NICE) Collaborating Centre reviewed the evidence on caries risk in relation to recall frequency, leading to the issue in 2004 of *Dental Recall: Recall Interval Between Routine Dental Examinations*.[1] Readers should refer to this guidance for an updated check-list for assessing caries risk in relation to recall frequency.

4.2 Children

In the diagnosis of caries in children, the weight of expert opinion supports the statement that posterior bitewing radiographs are an essential adjunct to clinical examination.[2R-5R] (One review[3R] has been classified independently by SIGN as a meta-analysis.) It has also become apparent that not only is the bitewing radiograph necessary for approximal caries detection, but that it can also offer a significant yield in the detection of occlusal caries.[4R-6R] The periodic bitewing examination can contribute to an individual's care plan for preventive and operative dental care. Information about lesion behaviour (progression, arrest, regression) can be added to a caries status assessment made at a first visit, and contribute to an appraisal of the patient's response to preventive therapy.

Although there is a need to ensure that radiographic exposures are kept as low as reasonably possible, this concern must be carefully balanced against the ethical difficulties associated with failing to employ a diagnostic aid that has been shown to detect clinically important numbers of lesions that would otherwise remain hidden from clinical examination. Even when approximal contacts are open, bitewing radiographs have a role in identifying occlusal lesions.

The importance of a high quality, standardised technique, using film-holding and beam-aiming devices, and ensuring proper processing, cannot be over-emphasised.

A patient should only be exposed to ionising radiation in dentistry after a thorough clinical examination. This should include an assessment of caries risk, as high, medium or low. *Appendix 2* lists some of the many factors that a practitioner will consider in making a caries risk assessment. The importance of the individual factors will vary from patient to patient.

This assessment of risk is central to deciding when to take subsequent radiographs.[2R,5R,7R-9R] This time interval will vary widely but it should be specific to each patient. Although reliable risk assessment can be problematic, clinicians are particularly good at identifying high-risk individuals.

The taking of 'routine' radiographs based solely on time elapsed since the last examination is not supportable.[9R,10]

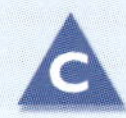

Intervals between subsequent radiographic examinations must be reassessed for each new period, as individuals can move in and out of caries risk categories over time.

4.2.1 High caries risk

Expert opinion supports taking bitewing radiographs at the initial examination for all children designated as being high caries risk.[7R,9R] In addition, there is a body of evidence to support this view.[11,12,13R,14-17]

There is a significant diagnostic yield associated with taking bitewing radiographs for use in conjunction with clinical examination for both approximal and occlusal caries detection, even in the absence of clinically detectable decay.[11,15,18,19] The amount of benefit is variously reported as being between 167% and 800% of the yield from clinical diagnosis, with or without fibreoptic transillumination assistance.

In terms of the contribution that radiographs might make to individual patient care plans, current evidence suggests that:

- If a small lesion is detected which radiographically appears to be less than half-way through approximal enamel, the lesion's location should be recorded and periodic review arranged. Preventive treatment should be instigated.
- If an approximal lesion extending to the inner half of enamel is detected, or if an outer half-lesion is seen to progress, preventive therapy should be instigated, and the results of such therapy should be periodically monitored.[7R]
- In a high caries risk individual, approximal lesions extending into dentine, detected radiographically have a great likelihood of exhibiting cavitation.[14,20,21]
- Additionally, it has been demonstrated that radiographic evidence of occlusal dentine demineralisation is significantly associated with heavily infected dentine;[22] therefore, the bitewing radiograph should contribute to operative care plans for such individuals with radiographic occlusal dentinal lesions.

It is recommended that all children designated as high caries risk have six-monthly posterior bitewing radiographs taken* until no new or active lesions are apparent and the individual has entered another risk category.

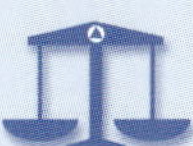  

** Bitewings should not be taken more frequently and it is imperative to reassess caries risk in order to justify using this interval again.*

It has been shown that in high caries risk individuals, lesions can still take up to 3-4 years to penetrate approximal enamel in permanent teeth.[23R] The time taken for caries to progress from the enamel-dentine junction to the pulp is unknown.[24R] Many authors consequently recommend six-monthly radiographs for high caries risk individuals until no new or active lesions are apparent. Radiographs should not be taken more frequently, and it is imperative to reassess an individual's caries risk in order to justify using this interval again.

4.2.2 Moderate caries risk

The evidence also supports the diagnostic use of bitewing radiographs for children with a moderate caries risk. Many authors report significant addition to the diagnostic yield from the use of bitewing radiographs, varying from 150% to 270% (the yield from clinical examination alone).[25-32] This increased yield relates to both approximal and occlusal caries.

Of the 12 studies in this area which passed critical review, no significant diagnostic yield was gained in three (in one study on four-year-old children,[30] in one where simulated clinical examination was supplemented by fibreoptic transillumination,[27] and in one when permanent teeth were clinically examined meticulously[33]).

On balance, the evidence supports the taking of posterior bitewing radiographs annually for children who are designated as being moderate caries risk.

It is recommended that all children designated as moderate caries risk have annual posterior bitewing radiographs taken until no new or active lesions are apparent and the individual has entered another risk category.

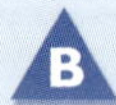

4.2.3 Low caries risk

Compared to that for high and moderate caries risk children, there is less evidence available to support the taking of posterior bitewing radiographs in children designated to be at low risk of caries. This may be due in part to the sample selection that many researchers have available to them, resulting in few studies in this area. The balance of the available evidence is unclear in relation to the need to take bitewings. Although the diagnostic yield from posterior bitewing radiographs is comparatively lower than that with higher risk groups,[34] high quality studies still show a significant yield, with estimates varying from radiographs revealing two to three times more carious lesions than clinical examination alone,[35] to 1.6-25% of clinically sound surfaces being found to have caries on radiographs.[35]

The evidence reviewed suggests that:

- In low caries populations such as Denmark, selective radiography should be conducted on surfaces suspected clinically as being carious.[35] There is continuing concern that hidden dentinal caries may affect significant numbers of low caries risk individuals,[36R] although there are a lack of high quality studies on the prevalence of hidden dentinal caries in low caries risk populations.
- In children with primary dentitions, the detection of three or more discoloured enamel lesions or dentinal lesions has been claimed to be a good predictor of there being additional dentinal lesions on radiograph, which could not be detected by visual examination.[37]
- In low caries risk groups, the time taken for approximal enamel lesions to progress through to dentine in permanent teeth is now in excess of 6-8 years on average and clinical decisions to restore must reflect this slow progression.[36R]
- There are particular problems associated with assessing sealed occlusal surfaces in low caries risk children; bitewing radiographs can provide a significant diagnostic yield, if used appropriately[38]

In the low caries risk category it is therefore all the more important for individual clinicians to apply risk-benefit calculations to each of their patients in order to make appropriate decisions.

It is apparent that the prevention-orientated child patient with little or no caries activity does not require bitewing radiographs at every recall appointment;[8R] however, it is very important at each recall to reconsider the child's caries risk status, as this may alter.

The weight of expert opinion supports the view that children at low caries risk should be radiographed at 12-18-month intervals in the primary dentition and at two-year intervals in the permanent dentition. More extended radiographic recall intervals may be appropriate if there is specific evidence of continuing low caries risk.[9R,24R]

It is recommended that children designated as low caries risk have posterior bitewing radiographs taken at approximately 12-18-month intervals in the primary dentition, and at approximately two-year intervals in the permanent dentition. More extended radiographic recall intervals may be employed if there is explicit evidence of continuing low caries risk.

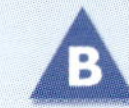

4.3 Adults

There is comparatively little evidence evaluating the present diagnostic yield of radiographs for caries in adults. It must be appreciated, however, that the carious process and caries activity are dependent upon interactions on a susceptible tooth surface of bacterial plaque with appropriate sugary substances, and these factors far outweigh a patient's chronological age. In the absence of experimental data from older age groups, it is reasonable, therefore, to extrapolate from the information available from studies of children and young adults.

There are particular reasons to be cautious in assessment of caries and caries risk in adults. As a consequence of the genuine overall reduction of caries prevalence across the UK population, when caries is present it often progresses very slowly and can present very late; thus cavitation into dentine may be visible for the first time in young adults who appear to be caries-free.

Similarly, caries risk assessments of adults must consider rapid behaviour and lifestyle changes that can have a significant dental impact. Changes in caries risk may follow the patient becoming less dextrous in plaque removal, a reduction in saliva following the use of some medications or the onset of

Sjögren's syndrome, and/or dietary changes following retirement, bereavement or a change in social environment.

Thus, while interpretation of the clinical examination and social history must be tailored to the age of the patient and the circumstances indicating the need for the clinical examination, the diagnostic benefits and limitations of dental radiography for adults are essentially comparable with those for children.

Root caries is an increasing problem for a minority of adults; although it may be prudent to consider root caries related to impacted third molar teeth (and distal surface caries in second molar teeth), there is comparatively little evidence in this area regarding radiographic selection criteria.

For these reasons, while suggesting that high quality studies with adults are needed, the same recommendations as made for children are made for adults.

4.3.1 High caries risk

It is recommended that all adults designated as high caries risk have six-monthly posterior bitewing radiographs taken* until no new or active lesions are apparent and the individual has entered another risk category.

** Bitewings should not be taken more frequently and it is imperative to reassess caries risk in order to justify using this interval again.*

4.3.2 Moderate caries risk

It is recommended that all adults designated as moderate caries risk have annual posterior bitewing radiographs taken until no new or active lesions are apparent and the individual has entered another risk category.

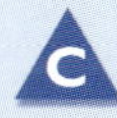

4.3.3 Low caries risk

It is recommended that adults designated as low caries risk have posterior bitewing radiographs taken at approximately two-year intervals. More extended radiographic recall intervals may be employed if there is explicit evidence of continuing low caries risk.

4.4 New radiographic methods and alternatives to radiographs for caries diagnosis

There is a considerable body of evidence relating to both children and adults looking at new methods and alternatives to radiographic caries diagnosis;[39R] however, this area is complex as the differing methodologies used confound direct comparisons.[5R,36R]

4.4.1 Digital dental radiography

There is a device which uses the transmission of laser light[40] and there have been recent advances in the use of electrical conductivity.[41,42]

4.4.2 Fibreoptic transillumination

For many years there has been debate in the literature about the potential of fibreoptic transillumination (FOTI), either to replace or supplement bitewing radiographs (*Figures 4.1-3*).[29,43R] The balance of evidence suggests that:

- It is an important adjunct which has considerable diagnostic value for detecting dentinal lesions at approximal sites.
- Bitewing radiographs will detect more dentinal lesions and many more 'enamel' lesions than FOTI (even though radiographs will still not detect all approximal enamel lesions).
- Research results with FOTI are obtained using custom-made 0.5 mm diameter tips in the hands of examiners trained in the use of this somewhat technique-sensitive method.

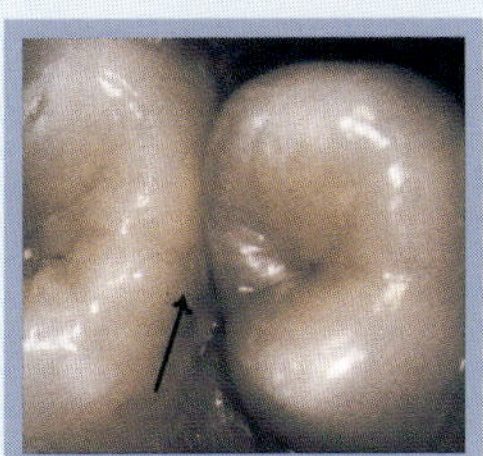

Figure 4.1 Clinically suspicious mesial surface of upper 6.

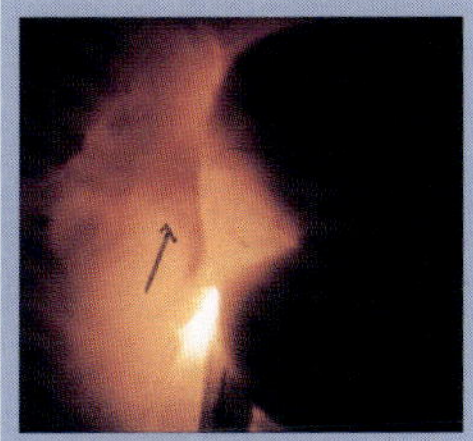

Figure 4.2 FOTI reveals a shadow within the mesial surface of the upper 6.

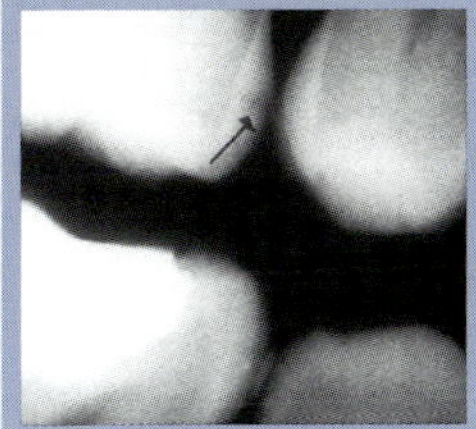

Figure 4.3 Part of a bitewing radiograph reveals a lesion in the mesial surface of the upper 6.

FOTI should be used as an adjunct to bitewing radiographs for caries diagnosis. When used, a 0.5 mm tip should be employed and training is recommended.

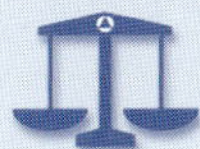

4.4.3 Elective temporary tooth separation

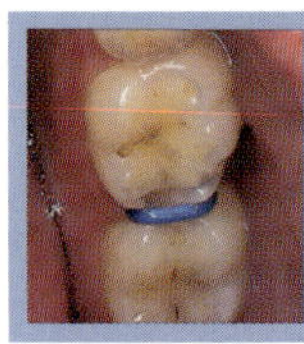

Elective temporary tooth separation (using orthodontic elastics between teeth) has been advocated[44] as a method of assessing directly the caries status of approximal surfaces. The method currently requires an interval of 3–7 days before the approximal surfaces can be viewed.[33,44-46]

It is particularly useful in determining whether or not cavitation has taken place.[21,46,47] Separation has been used successfully in Scotland, England, Brazil, Denmark and Sweden, and has been shown to be a viable tool in a general dental practice setting.[33]

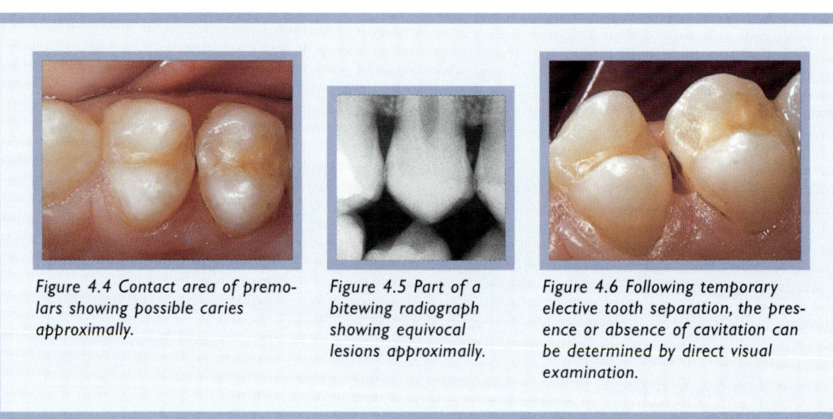

Figure 4.4 Contact area of premolars showing possible caries approximally.

Figure 4.5 Part of a bitewing radiograph showing equivocal lesions approximally.

Figure 4.6 Following temporary elective tooth separation, the presence or absence of cavitation can be determined by direct visual examination.

Consideration should be given to temporarily separating approximal surfaces where there is doubt whether or not cavitation has taken place and thus whether a filling is indicated.

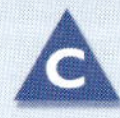

4.4.4 Electrical methods of caries diagnosis

Of the 'new' methods of caries diagnosis, there is a growing consensus that electrical methods provide the most promising results and the greatest potential for helping practitioners faced with the difficult task of diagnosing caries without using ionising radiation.[36R,48-50R] Although the commercial availability of simple systems is not yet widespread, this is a promising area where progress can be anticipated.[51]

The development and testing of electrical diagnostic aids should be monitored closely.

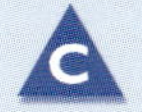

4.5 References

1. National Institute for Clinical Excellence (NICE) [home page on the Internet]. London: NICE; 2004 [updated 2004 April 8; cited 2004 May 11]. *Dental Recall: Recall Interval Between Routine Dental Examinations.* Available from: http://www.nice.org.uk/article.asp?a=112484

2. [R] Hanlon PM. Radiographic considerations in pedodontics. J Pedodont. 1985;**9**:285-301.

3. [R] Kidd EA, Pitts NB. A reappraisal of the value of the bitewing radiograph in the diagnosis of posterior approximal caries. Br Dent J. 1990;**169**:195-200.

4. [R] Weerheijm KL. Occlusal 'hidden caries'. Dent Update. 1997;**24**:182-4.

5. [R] Pitts NB. The use of bitewing radiographs in the management of dental caries: scientific and practical considerations. Dentomaxillofac Radiol. 1996;**25**:5-16.

6. [R] Henderson NJ, Crawford PJM. Guidelines for taking radiographs of children. Dent Update. 1995;**22**:158-61.

7. [R] Pitts NB. The bitewing examination as a preventive aid to the control of approximal caries. Clin Prev Dent. 1984;**6**:12-5.

8. [R] Howard HE. Rethinking pedodontic radiology. J Dent Child. 1981;**48**:192-7.

9. [R] Nowak AJ, Miller JW. High yield pedodontic radiology. Gen Dent. 1985;**33**:45-7.

10. Pitts NB. Score system for monitoring the behaviour of radiologically diagnosed approximal carious lesions. Community Dent Oral Epidemiol. 1985;**13**:268-72.

11. Stephen KW, Russell JI, Creanor SL, Burchell CK. Comparison of fibre optic transillumination with clinical and radiographic caries diagnosis. Community Dent Oral Epidemiol. 1987;**15**:90-4.

12. Stephens RG, Kogon SL, Wainright RJ, Reid JA. Information yield from routine bitewing radiographs for young adults. J Can Dent Assoc. 1981;**47**:247-52.

13. [R] Wenzel A, Pitts NB, Verdonschot EH, Kalsbeek H. Developments in radiographic caries diagnosis. J Dent. 1993;**21**:131-40.

14. de Araujo FB, Rosito DB, Toigo E, dos Santos CK. Diagnosis of approximal caries: Radiographic versus clinical examination using tooth separation. Am J Dent. 1992;**5**:245-8.

15. Creanor SL, Russell JI, Strang DM, Stephen KW, Burchell CK. The prevalence of clinically undetected occlusal dentine caries in Scottish adolescents. Br Dent J. 1990;**169**:126-9.

16. Nytun RB, Raadal M, Espelid I. Diagnosis of dentin involvement in occlusal caries based on visual and radiographic examination of the teeth. Scand J Dent Res. 1992;**100**:144-8.

17. Lussi A. Impact of including or excluding cavitated lesions when evaluating methods for the diagnosis of occlusal caries. Caries Res. 1996;**30**:389-93.

18. Ketley C, Holt R. Visual and radiographic diagnosis of occlusal caries in first permanent molars and in second primary molars. Br Dent J. 1993;**174**:364-70.

19. Wenzel A, Larsen MJ, Fejerskov O. Detection of occlusal caries without cavitation by visual inspection, film radiographs, xeroradiographs, and digitized radiographs. Caries Res. 1991;**25**:365-71.

20. Espelid I, Tveit AB. Clinical and radiographic assessment of approximal carious lesions. Acta Odontol Scand. 1986;**44**:31-7.

21. Lunder N, von der Fehr FR. Approximal cavitation related to bite-wing image and caries activity in adolescents. Caries Res. 1996;**30**:143-7.

22. Ricketts DNJ, Kidd EAM, Beighton D. Operative and microbiological validation of visual, radiographic and electronic diagnosis of occlusal caries in non-cavitated teeth judged to be in need of operative care. Br Dent J. 1995;**179**:214-20.

23. [R] Lervik T, Haugejorden O, Aas C. Progression of posterior approximal carious lesions in Norwegian teenagers from 1982 to 1986. Acta Odontol Scand. 1990;**48**:223-7.

24. [R] Elderton RJ. Assessment and clinical management of early caries in young adults: invasive versus non-invasive methods. Br Dent J. 1985;**158**:440-4.

25. Kidd EA, Naylor MN, Wilson RF. Prevalence of clinically undetected and untreated molar occlusal dentine caries in adolescents on the Isle of Wight. Caries Res. 1992;**26**:397-401.

26. Richardson PS, McIntyre IG. The difference between clinical and bitewing detection of approximal and occlusal caries in Royal Air Force recruits. Community Dent Health. 1996;**13**:65-9.

27. Mann J, Pettigrew JC, Revach A, Arwas JR, Kochavi D. Assessment of the DMF-S index with the use of bite-wing radiographs. Oral Surg Oral Med Oral Pathol. 1989;**68**:661-5.

28. White SC, Atchison KA, Hewlett ER, Flack VF. Efficacy of FDA guidelines for ordering radiographs for caries detection. Oral Surg Oral Med Oral Pathol. 1994;**77**:531-40.

29. Peers A, Hill FJ, Mitropoulos CM, Holloway PJ. Validity and reproducibility of clinical examination, fibre-optic transillumination, and bite-wing radiology for the diagnosis of small approximal carious lesions: an *in vitro* study. Caries Res. 1993;**27**:307-11.

30. Stecksen-Blicks C, Wahlin Y-B. Diagnosis of approximal caries in pre-school children. Swed Dent J. 1983;**7**:179-84.

31. Rimmer PA, Pitts NB. Effects of diagnostic threshold and overlapped approximal surfaces on reported caries status. Community Dent Oral Epidemiol. 1991;**19**:205-12.

32. Weerheijm KL, Groen HJ, Bast AJJ, Kieft JA, Eijkman MAJ, van Amerongen WE. Clinically undetected occlusal dentine caries: a radiographic comparison. Caries Res. 1992;**26**:305-9.

33. Rimmer PA, Pitts NB. Temporary elective tooth separation as a diagnostic aid in general dental practice. Br Dent J. 1990;**169**:87-92.

34. Ruiken HMHM, Truin GJ, Konig KG. Feasibility of radiographical diagnosis in 8-year-old schoolchildren with low caries activity. Caries Res. 1982;**16**:398-403.

35. Hintze H. Screening with conventional and digital bitewing radiography compared to clinical examination alone for caries detection in low-risk children. Caries Res. 1993;**27**:499-504.

36. [R] Pitts NB. Diagnostic tools and measurements—impact on appropriate care. Community Dent Oral Epidemiol. 1997;**25**:24-35.

37. Roeters FJM, Verdonschot EH, Bronkhorst EM, van't Hof MA. Prediction of the need for bitewing radiography in detecting caries in the primary dentition. Community Dent Oral Epidemiol. 1994;**22**:456-60.

38. Deery C. *An Evaluation of the Use of Pit and Fissure Sealants in the General Dental Service in Scotland* [PhD thesis]. Dundee: University of Dundee; 1997.

39. [R] Angmar-Mansson B, ten Bosch JJ. Advances in methods for diagnosing coronal caries—a review. Adv Dent Res. 1993;**7**:70-9.

40. Lussi A, Imwinkelried S, Pitts N, Longbottom C, Reich E. Performance and reproducibility of a laser fluorescence system for detection of occlusal caries *in vitro*. Caries Res. 1999;**33**:261-6.

41. Ie YL, Verdenschot EH, Schaeken MJM, van't Hof MA. Electrical conductance of fissure enamel in recently erupted molar teeth as related to caries status. Caries Res. 1995;**29**:94-9.

42. Huysmans MC, Longbottom C, Pitts NB. Electrical methods in occlusal caries diagnosis: An *in vitro* comparison with visual inspection and bite-wing radiography. Caries Res. 1998;**33**:324-9.

43. [R] Pine CM. Fibre-optic transillumination (FOTI) in caries diagnosis. In: Stookey G, editor. *Proceedings of the First Annual Indiana Conference: Early Detection of Dental Caries*. Indiana: Indiana University; 1996:51-65.

44. Pitts NB, Longbottom C. Temporary tooth separation with special reference to the diagnosis and preventive management of equivocal approximal carious lesions. Quintessence Int. 1987;**18**:563-73.

45. Pitts NB, Rimmer PA. An *in vivo* comparison of radiographic and directly assessed clinical caries status of posterior approximal surfaces in primary and permanent teeth. Caries Res. 1992;**26**:146-52.

46. Seddon RP. The detection of cavitation in carious approximal surfaces *in vivo* by tooth separation, impression and scanning electron microscopy. J Dent. 1989;**17**:117-20.

47. Danielsen B, Wenzel A, Hintze H, Nyvad B. Temporary tooth separation as an aid to the diagnosis of cavitation in approximal surfaces. Caries Res. 1996;**30**:271.

48. Ricketts DNJ, Kidd EAM, Wilson RF. A re-evaluation of electrical resistance measurements for the diagnosis of occlusal caries. Br Dent J. 1995;**178**:11-7.

49. Rock WP, Kidd EAM. The electronic detection of demineralisation in occlusal fissures. Br Dent J. 1988;**164**:243-7.

50. [R] Ricketts DNJ. Electrical conduction detection methods. In: Stookey G, editor. *Proceedings of the First Annual Indiana Conference: Early Detection of Dental Caries*. Indiana: Indiana University;67-80.

51. Longbottom C, Huysmans MC, Pitts NB, Los P, Bruce PG. Detection of dental decay and its extent using AC impedance spectroscopy. Nat Med. 1996;**2**:235-7.

Radiographs in Periodontal Assessment

5.1 Introduction

At present, there appears to be little direct research evidence from which to produce definitive guidelines for the use of radiographs in periodontology. In contrast, there is a very large base of periodontal research papers which include the use of radiography to assist in determining and confirming diagnosis, prognosis and monitoring of long-term treatment success. As these papers were insufficiently directed towards selection criteria, they were not included in this document.

The following points emerged from the papers reviewed:[1R-7R,8-10,11R,12-19]

- Diagnosis of periodontal diseases depends on a clinical examination, supplemented by radiographs where they may provide additional information which could potentially change patient management and prognosis.[4R,18,19]

- Clinicians should always use radiographs taken to assist the diagnosis of caries to aid their assessment of the periodontal hard tissues.

- There appears to be no evidence on when to take a periapical radiograph to assist in the diagnosis or treatment of periodontal/endodontic lesions.

- The use of computer-assisted densiometry without the inclusion of a reference object of known density and a highly reproducible positioning system is unlikely to be helpful.

- There is no clear evidence to support any recommendations regarding the frequency of radiographs taken for periodontal reasons.

- Radiographic assessment of changes in alveolar bone can be improved if sequential intra-oral radiographs are placed consistently to accurately reproduce 'the radiographic geometry'.[2R,3R,7R]

5.2 Conclusions from the literature reviewed

It can be concluded that the bitewing projection offers both optimal geometry and the fine detail of intra-oral radiography. Bitewings have the additional advantage that when they have already been indicated for caries assessment, they offer a means of providing information about bone levels around teeth without the need for an additional radiation dose.

While acknowledging that there is insufficient evidence from research into radiographic selection criteria for periodontology to make robust, evidence-based recommendations, the expert panel suggests the following.

If a patient has uniform pocketing <6 mm and little or no recession, horizontal bitewing radiographs are recommended.

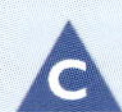

If a patient has pocketing 6 mm or more, vertical bitewing radiographs are recommended, supplemented by intra-oral periapical views using the paralleling technique at sites where alveolar bone image is not included.

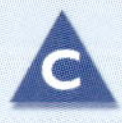

If a patient has irregular pocketing, bitewing radiographs (horizontal or vertical depending on pocket depth), supplemented if necessary by periapical radiographs taken using the paralleling technique, are recommended.

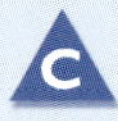

A panoramic radiograph of optimal quality may offer a dose advantage over large numbers of intra-oral radiographs and may be considered as an alternative, if available.[4R,5R,12,13] This may be the case when there are concurrent problems for which radiography is indicated, eg symptomatic third molars, multiple existing crowns/heavily restored teeth, and/or multiple endodontically-treated teeth in a patient new to a practice; however, in view of the limitations in fine detail on panoramic radiographs taken on older machines, supplementary intra-oral radiographs may be necessary for selected sites.[15]

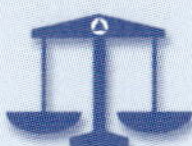 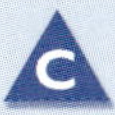

An intra-oral periapical radiograph using a paralleling technique is indicated if a periodontal/endodontic lesion is suspected.

 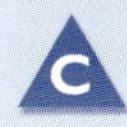

Members of the expert panel wish to emphasise that:

- The use of radiography should be viewed as secondary to a clinical examination in the diagnosis of periodontal diseases.
- Existing radiographs should be used as far as possible. Access to previous radiographs may be useful in assessing the rate of disease progression.
- Radiographs should only be taken for periodontal reasons after a thorough clinical examination has indicated their use as an adjunct.[1R,4R-6R,18,19]
- Radiographs can be important in helping to assess the prognosis of teeth affected by periodontitis, as they give additional information of root length and morphology (especially furcations of molar teeth) which the clinical examination does not provide.

5.3 References

1. [R] Absi EG. An evidence-based approach to guidelines in dental radiography. Postgrad Dent. 1996;6:26-34.

2. [R] Benn DK. A review of the reliability of radiographic measurements in estimating alveolar bone changes. J Clin Periodontol. 1990;17:14-21.

3. [R] Gutteridge DL. The use of radiographic techniques in the diagnosis and management of periodontal diseases. Dentomaxillofac Radiol. 1995;24:107-13.

4. [R] Hirschmann PN. Radiographic interpretation of chronic periodontitis. Int Dent J. 1987;37:3-9.

5. [R] Hirschmann PN, Horner K, Rushton VE. Selection criteria for periodontol radiography. Br Dent J. 1994;176:324-5.

6. [R] Stephens RG, Kogon SL. New US guidelines for prescribing dental radiographs. J Can Dent Assoc. 1990;56:1019-24.

7. [R] Wennstrom JL. Interpretation of radiographic data on longitudinal loss of periodontal attachment. J Periodontol. 1990;61:459-61.

8. Walsh TF, Al-Hokail OS, Fosam EB. The relationship of bone loss observed on panoramic radiographs with clinical periodontol screening. J Clin Periodontol. 1997;24:153-7.

9. Eaton KA, Woodman AJ. Evaluation of a simple periodontol screening technique used in the UK Armed Forces. Community Dent Oral Epidemiol. 1989;17:17-22.

10. Goodson JM, Haffajee AD, Socransky SS. The relationship between attachment level loss and alveolar bone loss. J Clin Periodontol. 1984;11:348-59.

11. [R] Jeffcoat MK. Radiographic methods for the detection of progressive alveolar bone loss. J Periodontol. 1992;63:367-72.

12. Molander B, Ahlqwist M, Grondahl H-G, Hollender L. Agreement between panoramic and intra-oral radiography in the assessment of marginal bone height. Dentomaxillofac Radiol. 1991;20:155-60.

13. Osbourne GE, Hemmings KW. A survey of disease changes observed on dental panoramic tomographs taken of patients attending a periodontol clinic. Br Dent J. 1992;173:166-8.

14. Rams TE, Listgarten MA, Slots J. Utility of radiographic crestal lamina dura for predicting periodontitis disease activity. J Clin Periodontol. 1994;21:571-6.

15. Akesson L, Rohlin M, Hakansson H, Nasstrom K. Comparison between panoramic and posterior bitewing radiography in the diagnosis of periodontol bone loss. J Dent. 1989;17:266-71.

16. Jeffcoat MK, Reddy MS. Progression of probing attachment loss in adult periodontitis. J Periodontol. 1991;62:185-9.

17. Rohlin M, Akesson L, Hakansson H, Nasstrom K. Comparison between panoramic and periapical radiography in the diagnosis of periodontal bone loss. Dentomaxillofac Radiol. 1989;18:72-6.

18. Tugnait A, Clerehugh V, Hirschmann PN. The usefulness of radiographs in diagnosis and management of periodontal diseases: a review. J Dent 2000;28:219-26.

19. White SC, Heslop EW, Hollender LG, Mosier KM, Ruprecht A, Shrout MK. American Academy of Oral and Maxillofacial Radiology, *ad hoc* Committee on Parameters of Care. Parameters of radiologic care: An official report of the American Academy of Oral and Maxillofacial Radiology. Oral Surg Oral Med Oral Pathol Oral Radiol Endod. 2001;91:498-511.

Radiographs in the Heavily Restored Dentition

6.1 Introduction

In the UK there are many individuals with a heavily restored dentition. The average dentate adult has seven filled teeth, but adults over 45 years of age have half of their teeth filled or crowned. Thirty-four per cent of UK adults have at least one crown, with 5% having six or more.[1] With restorations come the risks of dental caries, periodontal, pulpal and periapical diseases.

6.2 Diagnostic and treatment planning radiographs for new patients

Radiographs should only be taken if necessary for the diagnosis, treatment or prevention of disease. A thorough history and oral examination should always be completed prior to any radiographic examination.

> For patients with heavily restored teeth, posterior bitewings should be taken as recommended in Section 4, 'Radiographs in Dental Caries Diagnosis'.

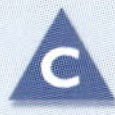

Information about a number of features of a tooth is required to plan treatment such as crown or bridgework. This includes such features as:

- Presence of caries.
- Condition of existing restorations.
- Level of bone support.
- Root morphology.
- Size of the pulp chamber.
- Signs of periapical pathology.

A number of these features may be evident from clinical examination or from bitewing radiographs, but others will only be evident on a periapical radiograph. Various selection criteria for periapical radiography have been suggested and subsequently validated.[2-5] Research has shown that the use of selective periapical radiography will give a high diagnostic yield. A flow chart, incorporating radiographic selection criteria, suitable for new patients presenting with heavily restored dentitions,[6] is shown in *Figure 6.1*.

When high yield selection criteria have already been applied, radiographs taken prior to crown or bridgework are very unlikely to yield positive apical findings. However, before preparing any tooth for a crown or bridge retainer

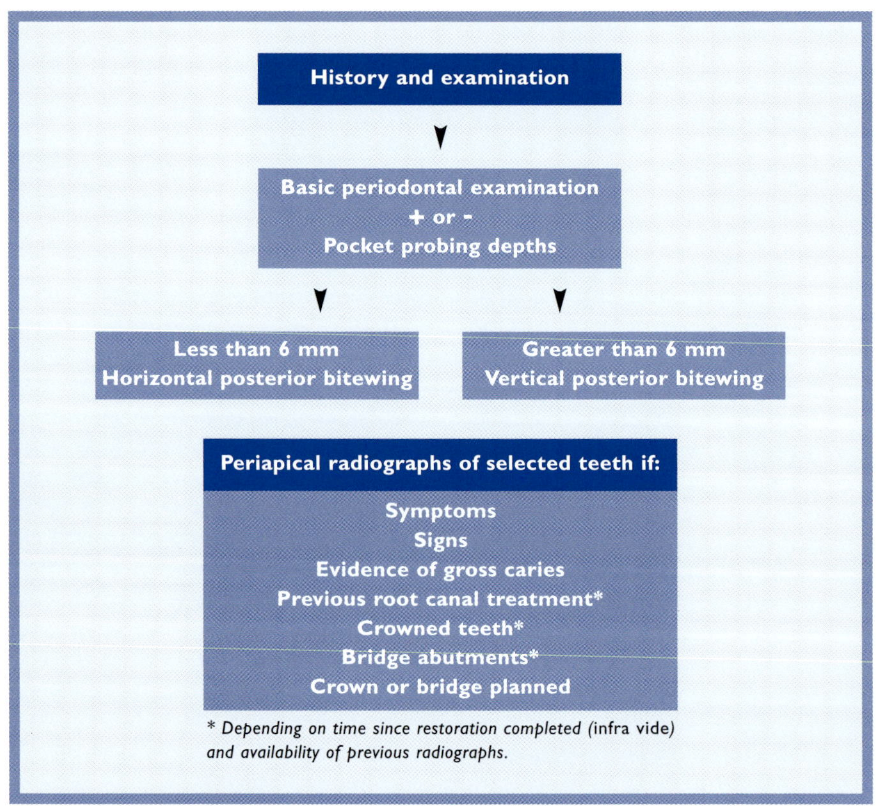

Figure 6.1 Initial radiographic examination for a dentate or partially dentate patient.

(conventional or resin-retained) or as a denture abutment, a periapical radiograph should be available as it will give baseline information about a number of features of that tooth such as the size of the pulp chamber or the root morphology.

Before preparing any tooth for a crown or bridge retainer or as a denture abutment, a periapical radiograph should be available, as it will give baseline information.

 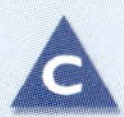

All radiographs should be taken using a beam-aiming device.

   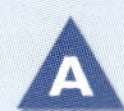

6.3 Follow-up radiographs of crowned teeth

For patients with heavily restored teeth, posterior bitewings should be taken as recommended in Section 4, 'Radiographs in Dental Caries Diagnosis'.

 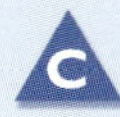

Histological studies demonstrate pulp reactions to dental treatment. There are many factors that have been shown to influence the loss of vitality of a crowned tooth. These include the pre-operative condition of the tooth, the cutting temperature and duration of preparation, the use of local anaesthetic and retraction cord, the length of time of temporisation, and the size of exposed root surface. The incidence and risk period of pulp deterioration following crown preparation remain uncertain, as a number of cross-sectional clinical studies have shown differing results. The approximate mean value for periapical changes on teeth restored with crowns and bridges is 10% at ten years.[7R] A longitudinal study showed 10% of teeth had pulpal deterioration over 25 years (mainly in upper molars and lower posterior teeth), with most pulp deteriorations being recorded after 2–7 years.[7R] Radiographic review before two years and beyond ten years post-cementation would be unlikely to give a high yield of radiographic findings.

Follow-up periapical radiographs of symptomless, vital teeth that have been crowned or used as bridge abutments are more likely to give positive apical findings if taken in the 2-10 years post-cementation.

  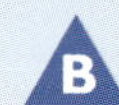

6.4 Follow-up radiographs of root-filled teeth

Where a crowned tooth or bridge abutment is root-filled, the guidelines regarding review radiographs recommended in Section 7, 'Radiographs in Endodontics', should be considered. Current research suggests that radiographic follow-up to root canal treatment at one year only is adequate in the absence of symptoms.

  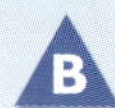

6.5 Follow-up radiographs of teeth restored with posts

Teeth that have been root–filled and subsequently restored with posts have a higher failure rate than root–filled teeth restored with crowns only.[8] Failure has been associated with reduction of the root filling to less than 3 mm.[9] Posts also present a risk for failure from root fracture and root perforation.

6.6 References

1. Pine CM, Pitts NB, Steele JG, Nunn JN, Treasure E. Dental restorations in adults in the UK in 1998 and implications for the future. Br Dent J. 2001;**190**:4-8.

2. Brooks SL. A study of selection criteria for intraoral dental radiography. Oral Surg Oral Med Oral Pathol 1986;**62**:234-9.

3. Akerblom A, Rohlin M, Hasselgren G. Individualised restricted intraoral radiography versus full-mouth radiography in the detection of periradicular lesions. Swed Dent J. 1988;**12**:151-9.

4. Brooks SL, Cho SY. Validation of a specific selection criterion for dental periapical radiography. Oral Surg Oral Med Oral Pathol. 1993;**75**:383-6.

5. Richardson PS. Selective periapical radiology compared to panoramic screening. Prim Dent Care. 1997;**4**:95-9.

6. Shelley AM. Dental radiographs. The Bridge Magazine (BUPA Dental Cover) 2000; Issue 19:14.

7. [R] Valderhaug J, Jokstad A, Ambjornsen E, Norheim PW. Assessment of the periapical and clinical status of crowned teeth over 25 years. J Dent. 1997;**25**:97-105.

8. Saunders WP, Saunders EM, Sadiq J, Cruickshank E. Technical standard of root canal treatment in an adult Scottish sub-population. Br Dent J. 1997;**182**:382-6.

9. Kvist T, Rydin E, Reit C. The relative frequency of periapical lesions in teeth with root canal-retained posts. J Endod. 1989;**15**:578-80.

Radiographs in Endodontics

7.1 Introduction

Radiographs are essential for endodontic treatment. It is possible to argue that endodontic diagnosis could be carried out without recourse to radiographs; however, it is not possible to carry out the mechanistic phase of treatment adequately without thorough prior knowledge of the root canal configuration and final confirmation that treatment goals have been achieved. The development of reliable electronic apex locators has greatly assisted in the provision of endodontic treatment.

Given that some radiographs are essential, it is important that each radiograph should provide the maximum diagnostic yield. This is achieved by:

- Ensuring correct exposure, handling and storage of the film.
- Using a long cone parallel technique, with the aid of a beam-aiming device.
- Using magnification when viewing films.
- Using a good quality, even light source for viewing, with masking of film from surrounding light.

7.2 Endodontic diagnosis

A thorough history of the complaint and a good clinical examination will often produce information to formulate a diagnosis. Review of the literature shows inconsistent evidence about the strength of the relationship between clinically observed signs and symptoms, and pulpal or advanced periapical pathology.[1,2R,3] A good quality pre-operative radiograph will give valuable additional information[4] for the diagnosis. At least one pre-operative radiograph is required for the next phase; therefore, there should always be a good quality radiograph available to assist in diagnosis.

7.3 Root canal treatment planning

Root canal treatment can only be justified if the tooth has a reasonable chance of being maintained in function for a significant period or if the tooth is essential for aesthetics. A pre-operative radiograph will reveal possible complicating factors such as severe periodontal bone loss, internal or external resorption, unfavourable root morphology, root fractures or other pathology. These may be absolute contra-indications to root canal treatment and, therefore, a radiograph will be an essential aid to treatment planning.

7.3.1 Non-surgical root canal treatment

If the decision is made to treat the tooth, a pre-operative film may give the following essential information:

- Form and extent of the coronal pulp.
- Number of roots of the tooth.
- Approximate length of the roots.
- Degree of curvature of any roots.
- Root canal morphology.
- Angulation of the roots.
- Degree of sclerosis of the root canals.
- Proximity of other anatomical structures (inferior dental canal, maxillary antrum).
- An assessment of the periradicular disease.
- Possible evidence of lateral or furcation canals.
- Evidence of previous endodontic treatment, pins or posts.

A pre-operative radiograph also becomes an important part of a patient's records.

In some circumstances, it may be necessary to take two pre-operative radiographs to reveal enough information.[4] In these cases, one film should be taken using a parallel-aligning device and another from a mesial or distal angle.

7.3.2 Surgical root canal treatment

Most of the above will apply to cases which require endodontic surgery because surgery is rarely considered until orthograde techniques have been properly excluded.

When evaluating a tooth for periradicular surgery, the following points must be very carefully considered when viewing the radiograph:

- The likely final length of the root with respect to periodontal support.
- The proximity of other anatomical structures.
- Evidence of root fracture.
- Presence of perforation.
- Evidence of lateral canals.
- The length of root filling apically in relation to the root length.
- Presence of extruded obturation material.
- The size of the periapical lesion.

Radiography for periradicular surgical planning should show an area of periradicular bone consistent with the extent of the likely surgical intervention. While a periapical radiograph may be satisfactory, larger images (eg occlusal radiographs) may need to be used as supplements to the periapical film.

> A good quality pre-operative radiograph is mandatory for surgical endodontic treatment planning.

 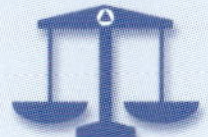 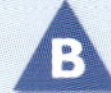

7.4 Root canal treatment

The aim of root canal treatment is to clean and shape the root canal system and then fill the space, densely, with a non-toxic obturation material. Traditionally, radiographs have been used in an attempt to check that the entire system has been instrumented and that instruments have been confined to the root canal system. In the absence of reliable electronic apex-locating devices, this is still the only method available.

Under certain conditions it may be necessary to take two (or more) radiographs in order to determine lengths of all the root canals (*Figures 7.1 and 7.2*).[5] In addition, if the diagnostic file is more than 3 mm from the radiograph apex, it is advisable to reset the file to greater length and take a second radiograph.

At least one good radiograph is necessary to determine working length(s).

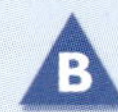

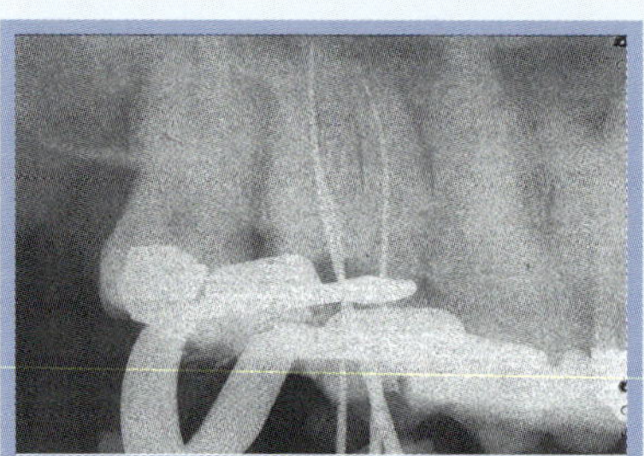

Figure 7.1 *This view of an upper second molar shows palatal and mesiobuccal roots clearly but the distobuccal root is obscured.*

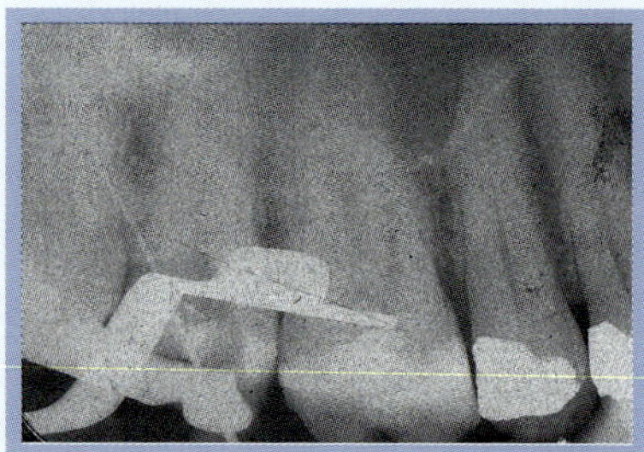

Figure 7.2 *A second radiograph of the same tooth. The angulation is different (the same effect may be achieved by altering centering of the beam) and the mesiobuccal and palatal files are removed. The unfortunate result is now clear.*

It is desirable for the filling technique to confine the obturation material to within the root canal.[6,7] Many operators recommend a radiograph to check progression of the obturation. Often termed a mid–fill radiograph, this consists of the chosen master gutta–percha cone with a small number of accessory cones condensed around it. It may depend on the chosen method of preparation and obturation, and the 'feel' of the apical stop. If there is any doubt about the integrity of the apical area, a check should be made.

> If there is any doubt about the integrity of the apical constriction, a mid-fill radiograph should be taken to confirm that the position of the cones before final condensation is carried out.

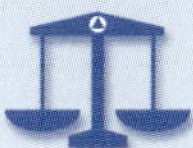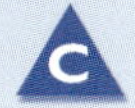

The latest multi-frequency electronic apex locators are generally very reliable at locating the end of a root canal.[8] They are also particularly useful for locating perforations.[9] The manufacturers of these devices continue to report that they are unreliable in certain circumstances, which include when there is too much fluid in the canals, when there is a large restoration present and when the apical foramen is large or damaged.

7.5 Endodontic follow-up

A radiograph should be taken immediately following obturation, using the paralleling technique and a beam-aiming device. If it proved necessary to take radiographs from additional angles to determine the lengths of the canals, it may be necessary to take additional post-operative radiographs for the same reasons. These radiographs should be processed and inspected before the patient leaves the surgery.

An immediate post-operative radiograph(s) will help in:

- A basic (two-dimensional) assessment of the quality of the obturation (voids in the material, apical extrusion etc).
- A baseline measurement of the apical state for follow-up.
- Consideration of possible complicating factors, such as apical 'zipping' or 'transportation', or potentially weakened areas of the tooth root due to over-preparation.
- Assessment of the best method for tooth restoration. Factors such as post length, type and diameter may be considered or deemed to be contra-indicated after reference to a radiograph.

At least one post-operative radiograph is necessary to assess the success of the obturation and to act as a baseline for assessment of apical pathology or healing.

The ideal follow-up for assessing healing has not yet been agreed. Studies have demonstrated clear signs of healing on radiographs at three months[10] and have suggested that the peak incidence of both healing and emerging chronic apical periodontitis is at one year.[11] Healing can continue to take place for up to four years and can be reversed if there is disruption of the coronal seal. A one-year follow-up is recommended to assess healing; if there is incomplete healing, a further annual follow-up is recommended until healing occurs. An increase in size of a lesion at any time or failure of a lesion to reduce in size after four years is usually a sign that treatment has failed.

Teeth that remain symptomatic may require additional radiographic review to assess the treatment options.

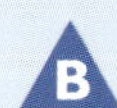

A further follow-up radiograph should be taken at one year after completion of treatment, even for asymptomatic teeth. Large periapical radiolucencies should be monitored more frequently.[12R]

7.6 Other endodontic treatments

7.6.1 Vital pulp procedures

Pulp-capping procedures and pulp amputations are performed in order to keep all or part of the pulp vital. Radiographic review is required to look for signs of continuing vitality or periapical pathology but this must be part of a complete clinical review. Signs of success on the radiograph may be formation of dentine (calcific) bridges and continued root development where it was incomplete at the time of operation.

A radiograph is necessary at the time of operation to provide information for treatment planning and to act as a baseline for evaluation of the procedure. Evidence of success would be expected at six months and this is the most appropriate time for the first review radiograph. Further annual review radiographs should be taken until root formation is complete. If the tooth is symptomatic or clinical signs of failure are detected, radiographs may be required as part of necessary treatment.

A baseline radiograph is essential for treatment planning in vital pulp procedures.

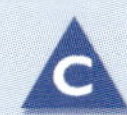

Follow-up radiographs should be taken at six months after treatment and then annually until root formation is complete.

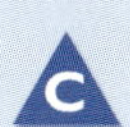

7.6.2 Trauma

Traumatised teeth require careful review, clinical and often radiographic. A baseline radiograph following the incident is mandatory. Ideally, this should be taken at the first visit, providing patient cooperation can be gained. A baseline intra-oral radiograph is mandatory following all but minor tooth trauma. If a diagnosis of root fracture is a clinical possibility, then two intra-oral radiographs taken from different angulations will be helpful in improving diagnostic confidence.

All radiographs should be taken using the paralleling technique with a beam-aiming device; this allows a degree of reproducibility.

Baseline radiography is mandatory following all but minor tooth trauma.

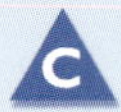

While all expert opinion supports the taking of review radiographs, there is no evidence to support any particular frequency or duration of review.

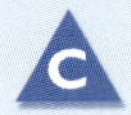

7.7 Digital radiographic imaging[13R]

Recent advances in this field have resulted in reliable machines at a reasonably affordable price. The images produced can be high quality and may be archived. They have the advantage of being able to undergo image manipulation, such as enlargement of key areas and change of contrast.

7.7.1 Possible advantages

- Potential for lower x-ray exposure.
- Images of acceptable quality, which can be manipulated.
- Very short time to view image on screen, and no chemical processing.

7.7.2 Possible disadvantages

- Possibility of not taking advantage of dose reduction potential.
- Increased reject rate due to problems in sensor positioning.
- Initial expense of equipment.
- While the ability to manipulate images may cast doubt on the medicolegal validity of digital images, archiving of the original image may address this problem.

Digital intra-oral radiographic imaging has some advantages over conventional film technology. It appears to give acceptable image quality and potentially can be used with lower x-ray doses to the patient.

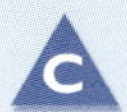

7.8 References

1. Krell K, Walton R. Odontalgia: diagnosing pulpal, periapical and periodontal pain. In: Clark J, editor. *Clinical Dentistry*. Philadelphia: Harper and Row; 1986.

2. [R] Chambers IG. The role and methods of pulp testing in oral diagnosis: a review. Int Endod J. 1982;15:1-15.

3. Dummer PMM. Clinical signs and symptoms in pulp disease. Int Endod J. 1980;13:27-35.

4. Klein RMF, Blake SA, Nattress BR, Hirschmann PN. Evaluation of x-ray beam angulation for successful twin canal identification in mandibular incisors. Int Endod J. 1997;30:58-63.

5. Fava LRD, Dummer PMH. Periapical radiographic techniques during endodontic diagnosis and treatment. Int Endod J. 1997;30:250-61.

6. Sonat B, Dalat D, Gunham O. Periapical tissue reaction to root fillings with Sealapex. Int Endod J. 1990;23:46-52.

7. Mattison GD, Haddix JE, Pink FE, Baughman R, Collins R. Periapical tissue response to root canals filled with Thermafil. J Dent Res, 1991;70:362.

8. Pratten DH, McDonald NJ. Comparison of radiographic and electronic working lengths. J Endod, 1996;22:173-6.

9. Kaufman AY, Fuss Z, Keila S, Waxenberg S. Reliability of different electronic apex locators to detect root perforations *in vitro*. Int Endod J. 1997;30:403-7.

10. Huumonen S, Lenander-Lumiken M, Sigurdsson A, Ostravik D. Int Endod J. 2003;36:296-301.

11. Orstavik D. Time-course and risk analyses of the development and healing of chronic apical periodontitis in man. Int Endod J. 1996;29:150-5.

12. [R] Consensus report of the European Society of Endodontology on quality guidelines for endodontic treatment. Int Endod J. 1994;27:115-24.

13. [R] Wenzel A. Digital radiography and caries diagnosis. Dentomaxillofac Radiol. 1998;27:3-11.

Radiographs in Implantology

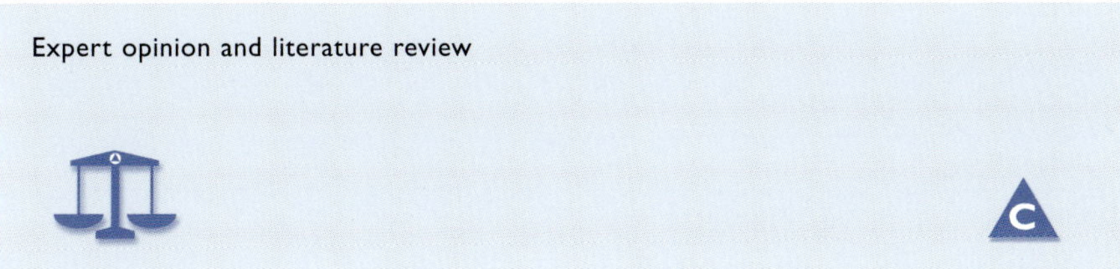

8.1 Introduction

In implantology, radiology plays a crucial role in treatment planning, the assessment of implant integration and reviewing implant function. Successful implant therapy is facilitated by the availability of adequate information about the quantity and quality of bone at the proposed implant site. Finally, radiology is needed periodically to assess healing and osseointegration.

The literature on radiology of implants was reviewed by a Medline search, examination of three review papers,[1R-3R] one consensus document,[4] a review of relevant sections of two textbooks on implantology,[5,6] and two textbooks of oral radiology.[7,8] From these, it was clear that there is considerable knowledge of the value of the various imaging methods used in implantology. With the permission of the publishers, Blackwell, two tables from the consensus document—the European Association for Osseointegration 'Guidelines for the use of diagnostic imaging in implant dentistry'[4]—are reproduced at *Table 8.1 (a and b)*. However, there was some disagreement on the selection criteria in individual clinical situations, and little information on the frequency and duration of follow-up radiographs after treatment completion. Overall, it can be concluded that, at present, there is a very small evidence base on which to formulate guidelines for the use of radiographs in implantology.

Table 8.1a: **Recommended standard radiographic techniques**			
	Intra-oral radiography	**Panoramic imaging**	**Cephalometric lateral skull**[†]
Maxilla			
Single tooth	X		
Partially dentate	X	X	
Edentulous	X	X	
Mandible			
Single tooth	X		
Partially dentate	X	X	
Edentulous	Axial, occlusal view[*]	X	X

* For Brånemark Novum cases only.

† Cephalometric wedge form collimation.

The Brånemark Novum Protocol for Same-Day Teeth; A Global Perspective.
Edited by Per-Ingvar Brånemark for Quintessence books in 2001.

8.2 Review of radiological techniques

Many radiological techniques are available to the dentist. The following are relevant to implantology.

8.2.1 Periapical radiography

Periapical radiographs are commonly used in implant therapy treatment planning. Apart from being the most appropriate method of assessing the remaining teeth and edentulous areas for pathology and the position of anatomical structures, periapical radiographs are often used to assess the bone height available. Following implant placement, they are particularly useful for assessing the success or otherwise of osseointegration, as their fine detail allows for the detection of small alterations in bone architecture. In cases where anatomical structures might limit safe implant placement, a stepwise approach may be adopted using a radiopaque instrument, placed to a known depth, sufficiently distant from the vital structure to allow safe further preparation of the implant site. The exact position of the radiopaque instrument is

Table 8.1b: **Recommended cross-sectional imaging modalities; special indications**

	Spiral tomography	Computed tomography
Maxilla		
Single tooth		
a. Incisive canal	1-2 x 2-mm cuts	
b. Descent of maxillary sinus	1 x 2-mm cut	
c. Clinical doubt about shape of alveolar ridge	1 x 2-mm cut	
Partially dentate		
a. Descent of maxillary sinus	Small areas (≤4 x 4-mm cuts per quadrant)	Multiple regions
b. Clinical doubt about shape of alveolar ridge		
Edentulous		
a. Descent of maxillary sinus	Specific sites targeted (≤4 x 4-mm cuts per quadrant)	Multiple regions
b. Clinical doubt about shape of alveolar ridge		
Mandible		
Single tooth		
a. Clinical doubt about position of mandibular canal	1 x 2-mm cut	
b. Clinical doubt about shape of alveolar ridge		
Partially dentate		
a. Clinical doubt about position of mandibular canal or mental foramen	1-4 x 4-mm cuts per quadrant	Multiple regions
b. Clinical doubt about shape of alveolar ridge		
Edentulous		
a. Severe resorption	1-2 x 4-mm cuts per sextant	Multiple regions
b. Clinical doubt about shape of alveolar ridge		
c. Clinical doubt about position of mandibular canal if posterior implants are to be placed		

then checked with a periapical radiograph. The position of the final implant placement should also be confirmed with a periapical radiograph.

The problems in the use of periapical radiography relate to practical difficulties in taking the images and in the limitations of a two-dimensional image. It is good practice to use film holders and the paralleling technique for all intra-oral radiography; however, this can be a problem when dealing with a resorbed edentulous alveolus, where the film holder may dig into the palate or lingual sulcus. The use of cotton wool rolls between the edentulous ridge and bite block may help; nevertheless, in some cases, periapical images may show little more than the superficial few millimetres of bone. A periapical radiograph gives no information about buccolingual bone thickness. It is this limitation that leads to the need for other specialised techniques.

All intra-oral radiographs are magnified to a degree dependent upon the focus/object/film geometry. A reference object of known size, in the same plane as the alveolus, can be helpful (in the same way as a length estimation using a file in endodontics). Radiopaque grids are available and these can be fixed to the film to provide a guide, but it should be remembered that they only show the dimensions of the magnified image, not true bone dimensions. As with all dental periapical radiography, rectangular collimation using a suitable paralleling technique should be employed.

8.2.2 Occlusal radiography

True occlusal radiographs, while having no role in maxillary implantology, may occasionally be useful in mandibular implant planning. The image may help to demonstrate the course of the inferior alveolar canal; however, the images only show the maximal buccolingual bone thickness, giving no 'feel' for the cross-sectional jaw shape. As with periapical images, magnification of images should be considered. *See Table 8.1.*

8.2.3 Panoramic radiography

Simple panoramic images provide good general information about bone height, the position of anatomical structures (such as the inferior dental canal, mental foramen and maxillary antral floor), and bone quality.

However, it is extremely important to remember that all panoramic images are magnified (by10-30%) and that such magnification may vary significantly at different locations within the same radiograph, depending upon the equipment used. Furthermore, positioning variations lead to changes in magnification,[9] along with distortion, which may vary considerably at differing points along the dental arch. As far as the latter is concerned, it is fortunate that vertical measurements are affected less than those in the horizontal plane. As a guide, during radiography it is useful to employ reference objects, such as ball bearings in a baseplate in the line of the arch over the prospective implant, as close to the proposed implant site as possible. At the early stage of edentulous patient assessment, leaving acrylic dentures in place will allow more accurate positioning of the bite peg. *See Table 8.1.*

8.2.4 Lateral cephalometric radiography

This may be of use in the anterior jaw regions because it gives a cross-sectional image of the mid-line of the maxilla and mandible. The view gives information on trabecular density of the bone and the potential inclination of any proposed implants in the region concerned; however, it is of very little use elsewhere in either jaw because right and left sides are superimposed. Care must be taken with patient positioning in relation to the beam, in order to reduce positioning errors.[10]

8.2.5 Digital radiography

A number of direct digital radiographic systems, both intra- and extra-oral, are available to clinicians. They have the advantages of rapid images and of allowing image manipulation to be performed. The facility to magnify images and carry out densitometric measurements may have particular use in implantology. The possible errors detailed in 8.2.1, 'Periapical radiography', apply equally to digital radiographs.

8.2.6 Cross-sectional tomography

This technique requires special equipment in which there is a controlled movement of the x-ray source and film around a fixed patient. There are two main types available. The first, using modified panoramic equipment, has additional software to allow cross-sectional images to be produced. This is relatively inexpensive but can be time-consuming and is a demanding technique for the operator to perform well; furthermore, variable magnification errors occur, similar to those that can be produced during panoramic radiography. The second type is a sophisticated x-ray machine primarily designed for implantology. It produces cross-sectional images of the jaws perpendicular to the line of the dental arches.

While magnification is—as ever—present, it is uniform and predictable in the case of more sophisticated equipment. It should be noted that using such equipment for multiple sites may result in a substantial exposure to radiation.[11] When employing tomography, it is recommended that an imaging stent, containing radiopaque reference markers, is used. The reference marker should be smaller than the thickness of the tomographic image layer.

8.2.7 Computed tomography (CT)

CT scanning is an imaging modality that allows the clinician to acquire sectional detail of the mandible and maxilla in a single procedure. To prevent excessive radiation exposure to the eyes and thyroid gland, a series of axial slices are captured and processed by computer to construct cross-sectional images of the jaws, often using dedicated dental software. The images may be made life-size, are normally accurate within a range of +/-1 mm, and can be reformatted to produce images in other planes. As the radiation exposure from CT may be considerable (*see Table 8.2*), the use of dose reduction techniques and limitation of the target field is imperative.

During CT, metallic objects—such as amalgam fillings—may cause significant artefacts, which can lead to difficulties in interpretation. While scanning times are fairly quick, any movement of the patient between successive axial scans will lead to image artefacts and inaccuracies in shape and size of the image.

8.2.8 Magnetic resonance imaging (MRI)

MRI is a sectional tomographic imaging modality that does not use ionising radiation. Direct cross-sectional views of the jaws may be made in any plane[2R]

<table>
<tr><td colspan="2">

Table 8.2: **Selection criteria for radiology in implantology**

TREATMENT PLANNING 

</td></tr>
</table>

Single implant

Anterior maxilla	Combinations of periapical, lateral cephalometric and panoramic radiography. Alternatively, use cross-sectional tomogram.
Anterior mandible	Combination of periapical, lateral cephalometric and panoramic radiographs. Alternatively, use cross-sectional tomogram.
Premolar maxilla	Combination of periapical and panoramic radiographs. Alternatively, use cross-sectional tomogram.
Molar maxilla	Combination of periapical, occlusal and panoramic radiographs. Cross-sectional tomograms may be particularly useful to image the morphology of the antral floor.
Molar mandible	Combination of periapical, occlusal and panoramic radiographs. Cross-sectional tomograms may be particularly useful to image the position of the interior dental canal and to show the concavity of the submandibular fossa.

Multiple implants

Combinations of the above become unwieldy in multiple implant cases, and the need for CT or MRI becomes more obvious; however, the radiation exposure in CT should be borne in mind.[13]

During surgery

Periapicals; consider digital systems

Post-operative

Periapicals and/or panoramic

Review

Periapicals and/or panoramic radiographs give good two-dimensional information but the surgeon must be aware of potential magnification errors. Cross-sectional tomography (or CT/MRI in multiple case) is appropriate in complex cases. The radiation dose to the patient should justify the technique employed.

All guidelines on frequency and duration of radiographic review appear to be the subjective opinion of authors. A review at 12 months is considered essential[3R] to assess marginal bone loss. Thereafter review intervals ranging from annual[6] to every three years[7,14] have been recommended.

It seems sensible to continue review until there is no perceptible evidence of continuing marginal bone loss, although review extending as far as ten years post surgery has been recommended as part of the basic criteria of implant success.

and with a high degree of accuracy.[12] The anatomy is best shown using T1-weighted sequences. Normal restorative materials are unlikely to produce significant artefacts on MRI scans. However, ferromagnetic objects, such as orthodontic brackets and temporary crown posts, can cause severe distortion. As image acquisition times may be longer than for other modalities, a good 'sequence design' is recommended.

8.3 Choice of techniques

An initial radiographic examination of a proposed implant site, using peri-apical films, is essential to exclude the presence of any retained root or other abnormality which might require preliminary surgery or contra-indicate implant placement. For assessment for bone quantity and quality, the selection criteria in *Table 8.2* are suggested. They must be used in the light of each patient's individual needs. CT is associated with considerable dose implications that need to be clinically justified. Cross-sectional tomography will give a lower radiation exposure when used in single sites, while MRI creates no exposure to ionising radiation. The choice of imaging modality may be limited by the availability of facilities.

Acknowledgement

Table 8.1 (parts a and b) is reproduced with kind permission of Blackwell Publishers, Oxford, United Kingdom, and was originally published as *Table 2* (parts a and b) in Harris D, Buser D, Dula K, Grondahl K, Jacobs R, Leckholm U, *et al.* EAO guidelines for the use of diagnostic imaging in implant dentistry. A consensus workshop organized by the European Association for Osseointegration in Trinity College Dublin. Clin Oral Implants Res. 2002;**13**:566-70.

8.4 References

1. [R] Frederiksen NL. Diagnostic imaging in dental implantology. Oral Surg Oral Med Oral Pathol Oral Endod. 1995;**80**:540-54.

2. [R] Gray CF, Redpath TW, Smith FW, Staff RT. Advanced imaging: magnetic resonance imaging in implant dentistry. Clin Oral Implants Res. 2003;**14**:18-27.

3. [R] Albrektsson T, Zarb GA, Worthington P, Eriksson AR. The long-term efficacy of currently used dental implants: a review and proposed criteria for success. Int J Oral Maxillofac Implants. 1986;**1**:11-25.

4. Harris D, Buser D, Dula K, Grondahl K, Jacobs R, Leckholm U, *et al*. EAO guidelines for the use of diagnostic imaging in implant dentistry. A consensus workshop organized by the European Association for Osseointegration in Trinity College Dublin. Clin Oral Implants Res. 2002;**13**:566-70.

5. Lekholm U, Zarb GA. Patient selection and preparation. In: Branemark P-I, Zarb G, Albrektsson T, editors. *Tissue Integrated Prostheses. Osseointegration in Clinical Dentistry*. Berlin: Quintessence; 1985.

6. Norton M. Dental Implants. *A Guide for the Dental Practitioner*. London: Quintessence; 1995.

7. Gratt BM, Shetty V. Implant radiology. In: Goaz PW, White SC, editors. *Oral Radiology. Principles and Interpretation*. St Louis: Mosby; 1994.

8. Whaites E. *Essentials of Dental Radiography and Radiology*. 3rd ed. Edinburgh: Churchill Livingstone; 2002.

9. Bolin A, Eliasson, von Beetzen M, Jansson L. Radiographic examination of mandibular posterior implant sites: Correlation between panoramic and tomographic determinations. Clin Oral Implants. 1996; **7**:354-9.

10. Verhoeven JW, Cune SC. Oblique lateral cephalometric radiographs of the mandible in implantology: usefulness and accuracy of the technique in height measurements of mandibular bone *in vivo*. Clin Oral Implants. 2000;**11**:39-43.

11. Dula K, Mini R, Lambrecht JT, van der Stelt PF, Schneeberger P, Clemens G, *et al*. Hypothetical mortality risk associated with spiral tomography of the maxilla and mandible prior to endosseous implant treatment. Eur J Oral Sci. 1997;**105**:123-9.

12. Nasel CJ, Pretterklieber M, Gahleitner A, Czerny C, Breitenseher M, Imhof H. Osteometry of the mandible performed using dental MR imaging. Am J Neuroradiol. 1999;**20**:1221-7.

13. Council Directive 97/43/EUROATOM of 30 June 1997 on health protection of individuals against the dangers of ionizing radiation in relation to medical exposure. L 180. Official J Eur Communities. 1997;9July:22-7.

14. Roos J, Sennerby L, Lekholm U, Jemt T, Grondahl K, Albrektsson T. A qualitative and quantitative method for evaluating implant success: a 5-year retrospective analysis of the Branemark implant. Int J Oral Maxillofac Implants 1997;**12**:504-14.

Good Practice

9.1 Do's and Don'ts

9.1.1 Do

Before taking a radiograph

In all cases:

- ✔ Complete a thorough history and examination, including the tooth-bearing areas.
- ✔ Seek originals or copies of radiographs taken elsewhere if they are relevant.

For caries diagnosis:

- ✔ Carry out a thorough clinical examination of clean, dry teeth prior to taking a radiograph (this may include transillumination, flossing, temporary separation of the teeth) and classify individual patients by caries risk category. (See *Appendix 2*: Selection criteria for radiographs according to caries risk status for children and adults.)
- ✔ Reassess caries risk status regularly (not only in children but also elderly and medicated patients). (See *Appendix 2*.)

When taking a radiograph

- ✔ Use the appropriate radiograph for treatment planning.
- ✔ Use F- or E-speed film for intra-oral films and rare earth screens for extra-oral films.
- ✔ Use film-positioning and beam-aiming devices for intra-oral films.
- ✔ Use rectangular collimation.
- ✔ Consider using a double pack radiographs if referral is likely.
- ✔ Report radiographic findings in patient's notes.

For all radiographs

- ✔ Ensure that processing conditions are satisfactory before processing a film.
- ✔ Ensure regular quality assurance in processing.
- ✔ Use an appropriate light box and magnifier for viewing, masking out any extraneous light.

✔ Mount, label and store radiographs appropriately.

✔ Follow national recommendations.[1]

9.1.2 Don't

✘ Carry out 'screening' radiographs or take radiographs as 'routine'.

✘ Take a new radiograph without examining existing films.

✘ Take panoramic radiographs for all patients.

✘ Use a single protocol for all patients.

✘ Use an inappropriate light source for viewing.

9.2 Ideas for audit—developing local guidelines

Clinical audit is a useful tool to check how well you and your staff meet the standards you set in your practice for almost any procedure. First, decide how you want to do something (set standards), and then look at how you are actually doing it (review practice). Next, compare the two and then make changes to your practice as appropriate (compare practice with standards and implement change). By repeating the whole process again, you can monitor your practice at regular intervals (known as re-audit).

Information needed to compare performance with standards can either be drawn from clinical records of patients seen in the past (a retrospective audit), or it can be collected from patients as they are seen (a prospective audit). The former relies on good record-keeping, whereas the latter allows you to make observations not normally recorded in the notes.

Simply setting new standards or guidelines and then expecting staff to adapt is not always very effective. Monitoring this period of change using audit provides the opportunity for feedback from staff about unforeseen problems and the time needed for people to modify their practice.

Details are given here of two ideas for audit. The first is about making good use of the resources in your practice, and ensuring staff follow best practice when taking, developing, storing and labelling radiographs. The second makes use of selection criteria for taking radiographs described earlier.

9.3 Audit of dental team participation in radiograph production

The aim is to ensure consistency in the quality of radiographs, while keeping radiation exposure to a minimum in both patients and staff. Many correctly exposed radiographs are rendered useless by poor processing, being lost or misfiled—which inevitably means repeat radiographs for patients. There are also medicolegal aspects. Radiographs must be kept for 11 years or until the patient is 25 years of age, whichever is the longer, and reporting radiographic findings in the notes is essential. (The counsel of perfection would be to retain records indefinitely.)

Thus, possible areas for investigation by the dental team are:

- Stock control of unused radiographs. (Is stock out of date? Is it stored correctly?)
- Taking radiographs. (Are they correctly exposed? Developed within a reasonable time? Were retakes necessary, and, if so, why?)
- Processing. (Were instructions followed correctly? Is equipment maintained?)
- Mounting, labelling, and filing. (Was it done correctly and in time for patient's next appointment?)
- Reporting findings. (Has this been done? How useful was it?)

Setting standards is a team effort, thus a preliminary discussion between members of staff responsible for these activities is essential.

Best practice can be agreed for relevant topics using resources such as the *Guidelines on Radiology Standards for Primary Dental Care*[1] (a 'quality assurance pack' has been produced from this document for dental surgeries), the British Dental Association Advice Sheet *Radiation in Dentistry*[2] as a guide, or manufacturers' instructions where relevant.

Guidelines can then be drawn up and displayed in clinical areas as a reminder. While these provide ideal targets to aim for, it would be unreasonable to expect 100% success or compliance even with the best of intentions and so in most cases it is necessary to set a lower, more realistic target such as 80% (for example 80% of all radiographs should be processed in time for patients' next appointments).

Finally, decide whether to review radiographs already taken (a retrospective audit), or look at ones as you take them (a prospective audit).

9.3.1 Example of a prospective audit

Collecting data: A list of things you need to know in order to measure and compare performance can be easily turned into a questionnaire, such as the examples given in *Figure 9.1*. Note that space is provided for additional

---

Figure 9.1 Sample templates for a prospective audit.

Patient ID	Radiograph type	Date taken	Exposure details	Date developed	Number of retakes and why?

A. Dentist/dental nurse to record when radiograph taken and processed

Filed correctly/ available at appt?	Mounted and labelled correctly?	Quality (contrast, position etc)	Can it be used?	Likely reason(s) for problem	Action required	Satisfactory report?

B. Dentist to record at patient's next appointment.

---

information (for example, reasons for retakes and problems with quality); these may be useful later. Decide who is going to collect what data, choose an appropriate method of sampling (for example, first 50 radiographs taken, or first 25 periapicals, bitewings and panoramic radiographs) and start measuring.

Analysing your data and comparing with standards: The aim here is to present your data in a way that allows direct comparison with standards (for example, the percentage of patients who had their radiographs developed in time). Once you know how staff performance measures up to standards, additional conclusions can be drawn about where problems occur most, using your comments to identify why things went wrong.

Making improvements: Present and discuss these results with the team and agree on action needed to improve performance eg change solutions more regularly, get developing machine serviced or buy a new one, staff training.

Re-auditing: To complete the audit, repeat the process at a later date to see whether practice has improved, changing your standards if they were too high or too low the first time.

9.4 Audit of selection criteria for taking radiographs

The care pathways chart (located at *Appendix 3*) summarises suggestions on how often radiographs should be taken to detect caries. These provide standards for the start of an audit.

9.4.1 Example 1

By looking back through patients' case notes, a very simple retrospective audit can be carried out, recording time intervals between radiographs in patients you have already seen (*Figure 9.2*). The results of an audit of this type only indicate what has been done in the past, possibly without any written guidelines. Also, information from patients' case notes is often limited.

9.4.2 Example 2

A more productive way of observing your use of guidelines might be to record what you do with patients as they come in, where you can make additional observations if you want to. Standards can be selected from the care pathways chart (*Appendix 3*) and other statements of good practice outlined earlier, and the audit used as a means of testing these out in practice—and, equally important, of seeing whether there are any problems using them

Figure 9.2 Sample template to record time intervals between radiographs taken to assess/reassess caries.

Patient ID	Time intervals between radiographs*				Other information relating to caries risk to help comparison with standards†			Caries risk status (high, moderate or low)
	Date last radiograph taken	Time interval (months)	Date previous radiograph taken	Time intervals (months)	Social history	Dietary habits	Plaque control	

* Add in more columns as required.   † Further examples listed in Appendix 2.

Figure 9.3 Questionnaire to record time intervals between radiographs taken to assess/reassess caries.

Patient ID	History and exam		Previous radiographs		Caries risk status		Date of next radiographs
	Completed?	Any problems?	Checked?	Any problems?	Assessed?	Any problems?	

Figure 9.3 is based on actions needed to assess correctly patients for caries. It almost serves as a personalised check-list for what to do, as well as a means to record problems experienced along the way. Far more inform-ation is available for collection, especially about why things go wrong; the information collected should make problems easier to solve. The check-list you use will vary according to the particular guidelines and treatment area in which you are interested, and, of course, performance and standards can be compared in the usual way where relevant.

9.5 More audit ideas

An initial audit may highlight areas worth investigating in more detail, or it may show up other problems not considered first time around. The focus of each re-audit can easily be tailored to meet the needs of the practice at the time. Some areas to consider are:

- Darkroom facilities.
- Radiographic image quality.
- Routine surveillance of equipment.
- Record-keeping of routine events and accidents.
- Daily evaluation of processing equipment using a 'test object'.
- Weekly checks on the number of radiographs taken.
- Protection for staff, and monitoring.
- Weekly checks on radiographic workload.

Recommendations have been published[1] for assessing quality of radiographs using a three-point scale (*Table 9.1*). These lend themselves to audit, and data analysis is kept simple. A more detailed look at reasons for poor quality could then be reviewed with re-audit.

<table>
<tr><td colspan="3" style="background:#2a4d9b;color:#fff">Table 9.1: Quality assessment of radiographs</td></tr>
<tr><td>Rating</td><td>Quality criteria</td><td>Targets: percentage of radiographs taken</td></tr>
<tr><td>1</td><td>Excellent—no errors of exposure, positioning or processing</td><td>Not less than 70%</td></tr>
<tr><td>2</td><td>Diagnostically acceptable—some errors of exposure, positioning or processing, but which do not detract from the diagnostic utility of the radiograph</td><td>Not greater than 20%</td></tr>
<tr><td>3</td><td>Unacceptable—errors of exposure, positioning or processing which render the radiograph diagnostically unacceptable</td><td>Not greater than 10%</td></tr>
</table>

9.6 References

1. National Radiological Protection Board (NRPB). *Guidelines on Radiology Standards for Primary Dental Care*. Report by the Royal College of Radiologists and NRPB. Documents of the NRPB: Vol. 5, No. 3. Chilton: NRPB; 1994.

2. British Dental Association. *Radiation in Dentistry*. Advice Sheet A11. London: BDA; 2003.

Overview of recommendations

t a history and clinical examination having been performed)

individuals		Endentulous
ESCENT	ADULT	
pecific radiographic examination consisting of posterior bitewings and periapicals. An extensive intra-oral radiographic examination may be ate when the patient presents with clinical evidence of generalised dental or a history of extensive dental treatment. Alternatively, a panoramic ph may be appropriate in some instances (see Section 2.2)		Periapical radiograph/s of any symptomatic or clinically suspicious areas
periapical or panoramic examination development of third molars if natic	Not normally indicated	
nonth intervals* or until no new or progressing carious lesions are evident ly and it is imperative to reassess caries risk in order to justify using this interval again		Not applicable
year intervals		Not applicable
year intervals. More extended radiographic recall intervals may be f continuing low caries risk		Not applicable
on consisting of selected periapical and/or bitewings for areas where pecific gingivitis) can be demonstrated clinically		Not applicable

Overview of recommendations (No radiographs should be taken witho[ut]

Patient category				Dentate
	SELECTION CRITERIA	**CHILD—PRIMARY DENTITION**	**CHILD—MIXED DENTITION**	**ADOL[ESCENT]**
NEW PATIENT	All new patients, to assess dental diseases, and growth and development	Posterior bitewing examination as indicated after clinical examination	Patient-specific radiographic examination as indicated after clinical assessment	Patien[t] selected appropr[iate] disease radiogra[phy]
RECALL PATIENT (See Appendix 2. Reassess caries risk at each visit)	Growth and development	Not normally indicated	Patient-specific radiographic indicated after clinical assessment	One-of[f] to asses[s] sympto[ms]
	High caries risk			Posterior bitewing examination at six-[...] *Bitewings should not be taken more frequen[t...]
	Moderate caries risk			Posterior bitewing examination at one[...]
	Low caries risk	Posterior bitewing examination at 12-18-month intervals		Posterior bitewing examination at two[...] employed if there is explicit evidence [...]
	Periodontal disease or history of periodontal disease		Patient-specific radiographic examinat[ion...] periodontal disease (other than non-s[...])	

Selection criteria for radiographs according to caries risk status

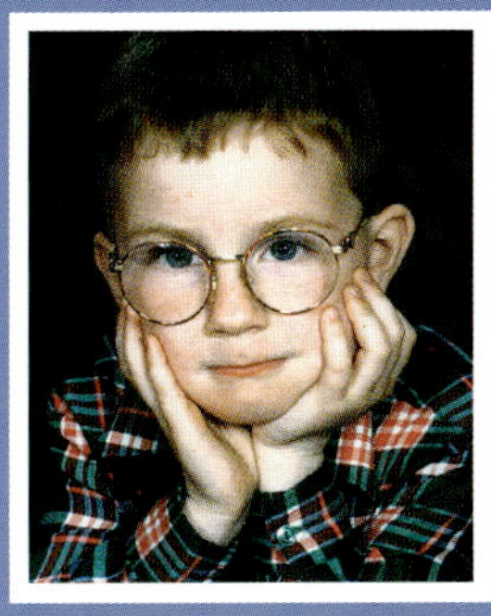

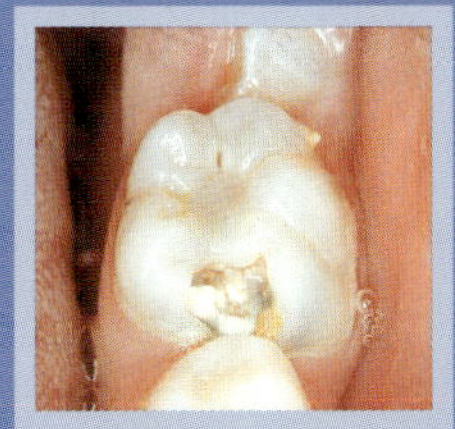

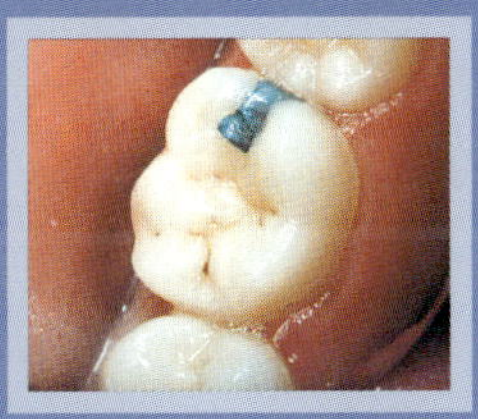

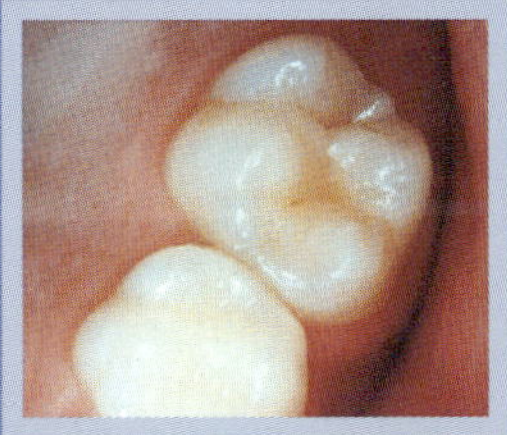

children and adults

CARIES RISK FACTORS

bits	Use of fluoride	Plaque control	Saliva	Clinical evidence
ugar	• Drinking-water not fluoridated[8R] • No fluoride supplements[8R] • No fluoride toothpaste[8R]	• Infrequent, ineffective cleaning[9R,10R] • Poor manual control[9R,10R]	• Low flow rate[5R] • Low buffering capacity[5R] • High *S Mutans* and *Lactobacillus* counts[11R,12R]	• New lesions, premature extractions, anterior caries or restorations, multiple restorations[11R,12R] • No fissure sealants[13R] • Fixed appliance orthodontics[14,15] • Partial dentures[16,17]

**OT CLEARLY FIT INTO HIGH OR LOW CARIES RISK CATEGORIES
AT MODERATE CARIES RISK**

| sugar | • Drinking-water fluoridated
• Fluoride supplements used
• Fluoride toothpaste used | • Frequent, effective cleaning
• Good manual control | • Normal flow rate
• High buffering capacity
• Low *S Mutans* and *Lactobacillus* counts | • No new lesions
• Nil extractions for caries
• Sound anterior teeth
• No or few restorations
• Restorations inserted years ago
• Fissure-sealed
• No appliance |

Risk category	Radiographic guidelines	Social history	Medical history	Dietary h[...]
HIGH CARIES RISK	**Posterior bitewing radiographs at six-month intervals* until no new or active lesions are apparent and the individual has entered another risk category** * Bitewings should not be taken more frequently and it is imperative to reassess caries risk in order to justify using this interval again	• Socially deprived[1R] • High caries in siblings[1R] • Low knowledge of dental disease[1R] • Irregular attender[2] • Ready availability of snacks[3] • Low dental aspirations[1R]	• Medically compromised[4R] • Handicapped[4R] • Xerostomia[5R] • Long-term cariogenic medicine[6R]	• Frequent s[...] intake[6R,7R]
MODERATE CARIES RISK	**Annual posterior bitewings unless risk status alters**		**INDIVIDUALS WHO DO N[...] ARE CONSIDERED TO BE**	
LOW CARIES RISK	**Posterior bitewing radiographs at approximately:** **12-18-month intervals in primary dentition** **Two-year intervals in permanent dentition** **More extended radiographic recall intervals may be employed if there is explicit evidence of continuing low caries risk**	• Socially advantaged • Low caries siblings • Dentally aware • Regular attender • Work does not allow regular snacks • High dental aspirations	• No medical problem • No physical problem • Normal salivary flow • No long-term medication	• Infrequent intake

References

1. [R] Beal JF. Social factors and preventive dentistry. In: Murray JJ, editor. *The Prevention of Oral Disease.* Oxford: Oxford University Press; 1996: 216-233.

2. Smith P, Nugent Z, Pitts NB. The burden of delay in seeking dental treatment in the Scottish GDS [abstract 395]. J Dent Res. 1996;**75**:1179.

3. Gustaffson BE, Quensel CE, Lanke LS, Lundqvist C, Grahnen H, Bonow BE, *et al.* The Vipeholm dental caries study; the effect of different levels of carbohydrate intake on caries activity in 436 individuals observed for five years. Acta Odontol Scand 1954;**11**:232-364.

4. [R] Shou L. Social and behavioural aspects of caries prediction. In: Johnson NW, editor. *Dental Caries: Markers of High and Low Risk Groups and Individuals.* Cambridge: Cambridge University Press; 1991: 172-97.

5. [R] Tenovuo J. Salivary parameters of relevance for assessing caries activity in individuals and populations. Community Dent Oral Epidemiol. 1997;**25**:82-6.

6. [R] Hobson P. Sugar-based medicines and dental disease. Community Dent Health. 1985;2:57-62.

7. [R] Rugg-Gunn AJ. Diet and dental caries. In: Murray JJ, editor. *The Prevention of Oral Disease.* Oxford: Oxford University Press; 1996: 3-31.

8. [R] Murray JJ, Naylor MN. Fluorides and dental caries. In: Murray JJ, editor. *The Prevention of Oral Disease.* Oxford: Oxford University Press; 1996: 32-77.

9. [R] Koch G, Arneberg P, Thylstrup A. Oral hygiene and dental caries. In: Thylstrup A, Fejerskov O, editors. *Textbook of Clinical Cariology.* 2nd ed. Copenhagen: Munksgaard; 1994: 219-30.

10. [R] Sutcliffe P. Oral cleanliness and dental caries. In: Murray JJ, editor. *The Prevention of Oral Disease.* Oxford: Oxford University Press; 1996: 68-77.

11. [R] Hausen H. Caries prediction—state of the art. Community Dent Oral Epidemiol. 1997;**25**:87-96.

12. [R] Johnson NW, editor. *Dental Caries: Markers of High and Low Risk Groups and Individuals.* Cambridge: Cambridge University Press, 1991.

13. [R] Gordon PH, Nunn JH. Fissure sealants. In: Murray JJ, editor. *The Prevention of Oral Disease.* Oxford: Oxford University Press; 1996: 78-94.

14. Zachrisson BU, Zachrisson S. Caries incidence and orthodontic treatment with fixed appliances. Scand J Dent Res. 1971;**79**:183-92.

15. Zachrisson BU, Zachrisson S. Caries incidence and oral hygiene during orthodontic treatment. Scand J Dent Res. 1971;**79**:394-401.

16. Yamaga T, Komoda Y, Soga K, Ono M, Asada T, Itosaka N, *et al.* Root surface caries of denture wearers in middle aged and elderly people. J Osaka Univ Sch Dent. 1994;**34**:65-71.

17. Drake CW, Beck JD. The oral status of elderly removable partial denture wearers. J Oral Rehabil 1993;**20**:53-60.